100 Questions & Answers About Communicating with Your Health_____er

John A. King, MD
(Retired Physician)

Cynthia R. King, PhD, NP, MSN, RN, FAAN
Special Care Consultants
Owner and Consultant

JONES AND BARTLETT PUBLISHERS
Sudbury, Massachusetts
BOSTON   TORONTO   LONDON   SINGAPORE

d Bartlett Publishers
ada
Sudbury, MA 01776
978-443-5000
info@jbpub.com
www.jbpub.com

6339 Ormindale Way
Mississauga, Ontario L5V 1J2
Canada

Jones and Bartlett Publishers
International
Barb House, Barb Mews
London W6 7PA
United Kingdom

Jones and Bartlett's books and products are available through most bookstores and online booksellers. To contact Jones and Bartlett Publishers directly, call 800-832-0034, fax 978-443-8000, or visit our website, www.jbpub.com.

Substantial discounts on bulk quantities of Jones and Bartlett's publications are available to corporations, professional associations, and other qualified organizations. For details and specific discount information, contact the special sales department at Jones and Bartlett via the above contact information or send an email to specialsales@jbpub.com.

The authors, editor, and publisher have made every effort to provide accurate information. However, they are not responsible for errors, omissions, or for any outcomes related to the use of the contents of this book and take no responsibility for the use of the products and procedures described. Treatments and side effects described in this book may not be applicable to all people; likewise, some people may require a dose or experience a side effect that is not described herein. Drugs and medical devices are discussed that may have limited availability controlled by the Food and Drug Administration (FDA) for use only in a research study or clinical trial. Research, clinical practice, and government regulations often change the accepted standard in this field. When consideration is being given to use of any drug in the clinical setting, the healthcare provider or reader is responsible for determining FDA status of the drug, reading the package insert, and reviewing prescribing information for the most up-to-date recommendations on dose, precautions, and contraindications, and determining the appropriate usage for the product. This is especially important in the case of drugs that are new or seldom used.

Production Credits

Executive Publisher: Christopher Davis
Associate Editor: Kathy Richardson
Senior Editorial Assistant: Jessica Acox
Production Director: Amy Rose
Production Editor: Daniel Stone
Associate Marketing Manager: Ilana Goddess

V.P. of Manufacturing and Inventory Control:
  Therese Connell
Composition: Spoke & Wheel/Jason Miranda
Cover Design: Kristin E. Ohlin
Printing and Binding: Malloy, Inc.
Cover Printing: Malloy, Inc.

Cover Credits
Upper right picture: © Monkey Business Images/ShutterStock, Inc.; Upper left picture: © Alexander Raths/ShutterStock, Inc.; Bottom picture: © dasilva/ShutterStock, Inc.

Library of Congress Cataloging-in-Publication Data
King, John A.
  100 questions & answers about communicating with your healthcare provider / John A. King, Cynthia R. King.
    p. cm.
  Includes bibliographical references and index.
  ISBN-13: 978-0-7637-5031-2
  ISBN-10: 0-7637-5031-X
  1. Communication in medicine. 2. Medical personnel and patient. I. King, Cynthia R. II. Title. III. Title: One hundred questions & answers about communicating with your healthcare provider. IV. Title: 100 questions and answers about communicating with your healthcare provider.
  R118.K56 2009
  610.69'6—dc22
                              2008028608
6048

Printed in the United States of America
12 11 10 09 08   10 9 8 7 6 5 4 3 2 1

Both Drs. King dedicate this book to their many patients and families who taught them so much, but also for the always constant love, support, and encouragement from Martha Remington King (wife of John and mother of Cyndy).

The current healthcare system creates many challenges and barriers for patients and their families. First, you must select a healthcare provider that you feel can meet your needs and then learn how to communicate effectively with him or her so that your needs are met. The question and answer framework of this book can guide you in how to achieve these goals.

You and your family members will learn how to break away from the traditional role of the passive patient of the past to become active participants in developing effective partnerships with your healthcare providers. You will learn how to:

- Select a primary healthcare provider so that you can become an active participant.
- Navigate the healthcare system more effectively.
- Use your limited time more efficiently with your healthcare providers.
- Stay healthy, prevent diseases, and optimize the care of your chronic diseases.
- Use online resources, associations, and foundations to enhance your health.

With support from your healthcare providers, you can take charge of your healthcare destiny.

Dr. Rick Botelho
Professor of Family Medicine, University of Rochester,
Director of Fellowship Training, Family Medicine Research,
and Fellowship Programs

Many books have been written about the difficulty in communication between individuals; by teachers to students; lecturers to groups; in families; and between married couples. It is not merely the words spoken, but includes the tone of voice, the mood, and gestures during the interchange, as well as the hearing of the recipient and the delivery of the speaker.

In the healthcare setting, some of the additional problems encountered are: fear on the part of the patient, lack of patience and/or compassion from the provider, prior difficult relationships with providers, preconceived ideas, or lack of focus by all involved during the meeting.

It has been said that many times two or more parties in a discussion arrive with their own agendas. With careful attention to what is being said, a few pertinent questions or comments, a great deal may be accomplished.

It is important for patient and provider to remember what the meeting is about and help one another to arrive at an understanding. From that comes a plan to make a firm diagnosis through examination, tests, and treatment. Depending on the complexity of the problem, it may require longer observation, further visits, consultation, and even hospitalization.

The main purpose of this book is to help laypeople communicate successfully with their healthcare providers (MDs, DOs, NPs, PAs). Communication must be a two-way road. The patient and family need to be good listeners just as healthcare providers need to be active listeners.

It is essential that there is effective communication between the patient and family and the healthcare provider (HCP) because the patient-physician relationship depends on trust and understanding of one another. This relationship must be a partnership. If the patient trusts the provider then he/she may be more apt to talk more freely and give more valuable clues to help the provider make the diagnosis. Additionally, the patient may feel more comfortable asking questions and eventually become more at ease with the recommended treatment. To feel more comfortable, you want to choose a provider that will sit down and listen, maintain eye contact, shows interest, be compassionate, and display concern.

In Part 1 of this book we will define the healthcare professionals who may care for you at your primary care physician's office (physicians, nurse practitioners, physician assistants, nurses, receptionist, secretary, and billing clerk). You may have other individuals involved in your care because of additional services you need (e.g., *home care*) or a recent hospitalization (e.g., *social worker*). After we define the healthcare professionals, the other parts of the book will focus on the key HCPs that can diagnose and treat you. These are physicians (MD or DO), nurse practitioners (NP) and physician assistants (PA). Because any one of these providers can treat you at your primary care provider's office we will use the term "healthcare professional(s)" or the abbreviation HCP throughout the book.

The majority of this book will assist you in taking a more active role in your health, especially by developing an open, honest, collegial relationship with your HCP. The questions and answers will help you to develop and maintain effective communication skills to use with your HCP. This will further help you to ask questions and negotiate treatment options.

PART ONE

Types of Healthcare Providers

What is the difference between an MD and a DO?

What is the difference between an NP and a PA?

Will registered nurses be a part of my healthcare team?

More . . .

1. What is the difference between an MD and a DO?

A **physician (MD)** is a licensed medical practitioner, a person who practices medicine, a person licensed as a medical doctor by the jurisdiction in which he/she is resident to practice the healing arts.

A **Doctor of Osteopathy (DO)** has a Doctor's degree in Osteopathy, which is a system of medicine based on the theory that disturbances in the musculoskeletal system affect other bodily parts, causing many disorders that can be corrected by various manipulative techniques in conjunction with conventional medical, surgical, pharmacological, and other therapeutic procedures.

2. What is the difference between an NP and a PA?

A **Nurse Practitioner (NP)** is a registered nurse (RN) with a master's degree who has completed additional courses and specialized training. Nurse practitioners can work with or without the supervision of a physician. They take on additional duties in diagnosis and treatment of patients, and in most states they write all types of prescriptions.

Physician Assistant (PA) is a trained, licensed individual who can diagnose, treat, and write prescriptions under the direction of a supervising physician.

3. Will registered nurses be a part of my healthcare team?

Your doctor may have one or more **Registered Nurses (RN)**. An RN is a nurse who has graduated from a formal program of nursing education (diploma school, associate degree, or baccalaureate program) and is registered and licensed by the appropriate state authority.

4. Who will be the other members of my healthcare team?

Some doctors have registered nurses and **Licensed Practical Nurses (LPN)**. An LPN has a two-year degree in nursing and is limited in the care they can provide under the direction of an RN, NP, PA, or MD.

Most offices have a **Receptionist**. The main duty of this individual is to answer the telephone, receive patients, check insurance, and check appointments. This is an office/administrative support position and is usually performed in a front office.

There also may be a **Secretary**. The secretary is an office/administrative support position. The title refers to a person who performs routine, administrative tasks for the doctor, NP, and/or PA. These office employees perform duties such as typing, computer processing, and/or transcribing dictation.

Becky's comments:

This viewpoint seems to center mainly on who your health-care team is when you are inside the doctor's office. Outside the doctor's office, there are two very important members of your healthcare team—your pharmacist and your insurance company. Your pharmacist is the one who explains your medicines—what they are for and how to take them. Your insurance company can help determine where you are seen for treatment and how you will be billed.

5. Who will help me if I have billing or insurance problems?

If the doctor's office is very busy, they may have a **Billing Clerk**. Medical Billing Clerks are responsible for compiling and maintaining records of the charges for services rendered at the healthcare facility. Once they calculate the total amount due from a patient, they must prepare invoices to be sent out and ensure prompt payment. Another major responsibility for a medical billing clerk is to contact insurance companies to determine what services will be reimbursed and for how much. Most medical billing clerks use sophisticated computer programs that allow them to calculate charges and print bills in one step. These programs also serve as a safety net because the biller has to verify the information that is entered and correct any errors before the bill is printed and sent to the patient. Other responsibilities may include handling follow-up questions from patients, resolving discrepancies or errors, and ensuring that all billing and accounting records are kept in a safe place.

PART TWO

Locating and Selecting a Primary Care Healthcare Provider

What type of healthcare professional should I locate for my general health problems?

What do I need to do before I start my search for a primary HCP?

What sources should I use to locate my primary care HCP?

More . . .

6. What type of healthcare provider should I locate for my general health problems?

In addition to MDs, there are, in some states, Nurse Practitioners (NPs), Physician Assistants (PAs) and Doctors of Osteopathy (DOs). For a family, a good choice might be a **Family Practitioner** who will care for all family members. An alternative to this could be a **Pediatrician** trained to take care of children and an **Internist** who provides care for adults. Women should also have a **Gynecologist** to take care of female health issues. If you are 60–65 years of age or older, you may choose to see a **Geriatrician**. There are many specialists whose practices are limited and come from referrals by the Generalists. Depending on state laws, NPs and PAs may practice from their own office or under the supervision of a physician.

7. What do I need to do before I start my search for a primary HCP?

The ideal time to select a new HCP is when you are well. For example, if you have just moved to a new city and you are well, you will have more time and energy to look carefully for a great HCP.

Also, before you start your search it is best to define your medical needs. Generally, when looking for a primary HCP you are seeking a long-term relationship with an individual who will oversee your medical care. What you are looking for may depend on your age, medical history, and personality.

Becky's comments:

It is important to examine characteristics of an HCP and how they fit with you. For example, a fifty-year-old woman who is in the early stages of menopause may feel most comfortable with a female doctor. By the same token, someone who prefers complementary medicine may want a physician who also prefers that approach.

8. What sources should I use to locate my primary care HCP?

Several sources are available to assist you in locating a Provider. The suggestion of a friend may be a good choice. There may be a local or a county Medical Association which may provide a list of names and specialties. A local hospital may also be a source. You may want to use the Internet and go to several of the websites listed in the Appendix (e.g., AIM Docfinder, AMA Physician Select, American Board of Medical Specialties, Best Hospital Finder listed in *U.S. News and World Report*). It may take more than one try to make the right match, but confidence in your provider is important. When making a first visit to a Provider, one is often asked to complete a questionnaire regarding health matters. This may include: a history of vaccinations, serious illnesses, operations, current problems, and medications. Taking all of this information with you, including dates in written form, will save time.

It may take more than one try to make the right match, but confidence in your provider is important.

Becky's comments:

Your insurance company plays a huge part in this! The manner in which it is handled often depends on your plan and coverage. Many insurance companies have a database for locating a physician that is covered by your plan.

9. What should I look for when selecting a primary HCP?

You should select a primary HCP in whom you trust and who will oversee your care. Your primary HCP should also be your advocate and guide you through the healthcare system. This individual does not have to specialize in everything, but should seek advice and consultation from other HCPs as needed. One of the most important qualities you want is an HCP who can communicate effectively with you. A good primary HCP should:

1. Take time to listen—and you need to help by explaining the problem clearly
2. Take time to talk to you and explain the treatment plan clearly
3. Plan ahead to help prevent health problems and future illnesses
4. Review your total health regularly
5. Have your trust and confidence
6. Be willing to let you ask questions and to give thorough answers
7. Have friendly, helpful office staff and adequate staff support
8. Respect your desire if you want a second opinion
9. Treat the "whole you" rather than just your physical symptoms
10. Be available by telephone—some simple questions can be answered on the telephone

You should select a primary HCP in whom you trust and who will oversee your care. Your primary HCP should also be your advocate and guide you through the healthcare system.

One of the most important qualities you want is an HCP who can communicate effectively with you.

10. Because effective communication skills are so important in selecting an HCP, how do I evaluate an HCP's communication skills?

Open, honest communication is the key to a true partnership with your HCP. In order to have a partnership or "collegial" relationship with your HCP you need to assess his or her communication skills. Communication skills come in several forms: written, verbal, and nonverbal. You can evaluate the written skills of your HCP by reading things he or she writes down for you or reading brochures they have created for their patients.

Communication skills come in several forms: written, verbal, and nonverbal.

It is often easiest to assess the verbal communication skills of your HCP. If your HCP has effective verbal communication skills you will experience some of the following:

- They will treat you with respect while you are talking
- They will make sure you understand everything they have explained
- They will use "lay" terms when explaining things rather than medical terms, and
- They will listen carefully when you are speaking or asking questions.

Lastly, nonverbal cues are also an important part of successful communication skills. Nonverbal cues include facial expressions, eye contact while you are talking, sitting down close to you, and nodding to agree with what you are saying.

Research has clearly shown that successful communication between a patient and an HCP can lead to better patient outcomes (e.g., better emotional health, better symptom resolution, better functional and physical status).

Research has clearly shown that successful communication between a patient and an HCP can lead to better patient outcomes (e.g., better emotional health, better symptom resolution, better functional and physical status).

If you cannot communicate with your HCP try another one. Sometimes two people just do not see eye to eye. But try to stay with one HCP for as long as possible so they can get to know you.

11. Is there ever a time when effective communication skills are not as important in the selection of an HCP?

You will still want the specialist to communicate with you, but you also want to pay attention to the technical skills of the specialist or subspecialist.

Medicine has advanced tremendously in the past 5 decades. Consequently, there is also a technical side to modern medicine. For example, someday you may need major surgery. In this case you will be selecting a specialist or subspecialist (this will be discussed further in another section of the book). The criteria you use to choose the specialist may be a little different. You will still want the specialist to communicate with you, but you also want to pay attention to the technical skills of the specialist or subspecialist. Ask the specialist how often they have performed the procedure you will be having. And make sure your primary care HCP has complete confidence in the specialist. You may want to see some before and after photographs or talk to other patients who have had the same surgery performed by this specialist.

12. Should I ask if my HCP is certified?

Although it is NOT required to practice, many MDs and DOs are "Board Certified." This means they have passed exams in a particular specialty. The American Board of Medical Specialties (ABMS) (Appendix) is the premier medical specialty certification board for MDs. Board certification means only that the MD passed the minimum standard of excellence at the time he/she took the test (usually at the beginning of his or her career). Nurse Practitioners also generally take a certification exam for their specialty (e.g., family NP, adult NP). Many of these exams are administered by an arm of the American Nurses Association called the American Nurses' Credentialing Center. You can ask your HCP if they are certified and in what specialty. But, they can still be an excellent HCP without being certified.

13. Is philosophy an important part of selecting an HCP?

HCPs vary widely on their philosophy of practice, which stems from their beliefs, opinions, values, and experiences. Most patients assume treatment plans are based only on scientific fact, but that is not true. Some HCPs may believe in treating patients "at all costs" which involves aggressive and invasive treatments. Additionally, you as an individual have your own philosophy, beliefs, and values. You may need to research your own condition to understand it or you may prefer to have the HCP explain it to you. Furthermore, you my NOT wish to have aggressive and invasive treatments, but instead prefer to spend time with family and friends and activities you enjoy. For a collegial relationship, you may want to have a similar philosophy as your HCP.

You can ask your HCP if they are certified and in what specialty. But, they can still be an excellent HCP without being certified.

Becky's comments:

It may be difficult to determine your HCP's philosophy right away. During your appointment, you may want to ask questions such as how he/she feels about end-of-life issues, the use of complementary medicine, or other things that are important to you in your health care. You may also get a feel for their philosophy indirectly through conversation.

14. What if I have a specific hospital I want to use?

If you have a specific hospital at which you want to receive all procedures, hospitalizations, and treatments, you will need to make sure to ask any HCPs you are interviewing if they can admit and care for patients at that specific hospital.

If there are several hospitals where you live and you do not care which hospital you are admitted to, then it will depend on where your HCP has "Hospital Privileges." Some HCPs have privileges to admit patients to more than one hospital. However, if you have a specific hospital at which you want to receive all procedures, hospitalizations, and treatments, you will need to make sure to ask any HCPs you are interviewing if they can admit and care for patients at that specific hospital. You also might want to check a website to locate ratings of hospitals (Appendix). One example is: Best Hospitals Finder (*U.S. News and World Report*) *health.usnews.com/sections/health/best-hospitals.*

15. What information should my healthcare provider know about me?

For physicians, NPs, and PAs to provide the best possible care for you, they need to know more than the facts of your illness.

For physicians, NPs, and PAs to provide the best possible care for you, they need to know more than the facts of your illness. Medicine is not an exact science, and several approaches may be equally appropriate. You need to be willing to talk openly with your provider and be honest. In order to decide your treatment, your provider may look at your particular case, you person-ally, your general philosophy about your health, and your ability to cope with illness.

Some of the following information may be helpful to your physician in the beginning:

- Your occupation and degree of physical exercise and mental status
- Close relatives who have had chronic illnesses like cancer
- Any chronic illnesses that you have
- How much you know about chronic illness and its treatment
- Degree to which you are affected by family problems, financial problems, work problems, or other difficulties
- Your hobbies, interests
- Your preferences regarding quality of life versus quantity life and whether you wish to be resusci-tated if your heart or lungs stop

PART THREE

First Visit with Your Healthcare Provider

What should I take to my first visit?

How will I remember everything I want to ask and everything that is described to me?

What will we talk about at the first visit?

More . . .

16. What should I take to my first visit?

On a first visit with a HCP it is important to have a clear idea what it is you want. A written note stating not more than 2 or 3 problems will expedite matters. It will be appreciated if you bring a written list of immuniza-tions, serious illness, opera-tions and any hospitaliza-tions.

On a first visit with a HCP it is important to have a clear idea what it is you want. A written note stating not more than 2 or 3 problems will expedite matters. It will be appreciated if you bring a written list of immunizations, serious illness, operations and any hospitalizations. It is also helpful to bring a legible past medical history as described in the Introduction and a current list of medications, or the drugs themselves in the bottle with the prescription label, as well as frequently used over-the-counter preparations (e.g., vitamins, herbs, cold or allergy medications). For instance, it is crucial to know if you are allergic to anything—medications, bees, foods. If you are pregnant or think you are pregnant, tell the HCP. If you have consulted other HCPs, bring those records or X-rays with you.

Nancy's comments:

Keep a list of all prior surgeries with approximate dates if you will be seeing a new HCP.

17. How will I remember everything I want to ask and everything that is described to me?

Many indi-viduals find it easiest to bring a notebook with a list of problems (limit to 1–3 if possible) clearly stated, with duration, previous tests, and treatment, including results.

Many individuals find it easiest to bring a notebook with a list of problems (limit to 1–3 if possible) clearly stated, with duration, previous tests, and treatment, including results. The notebook can also be used to record the diagnosis given by the HCP, any recommended tests, treatments, and medications. Be sure to have the HCP spell medical terms and prescription names for you and draw illustrations for you or give you photos. Ask about side effects to new medications and compatibility with any others you may be taking. The HCP may ask for other information. You may want to bring a trusted friend or relative if you are worried or uncertain about the occasion or want someone to help you remember what is said. Your family member or friend should be someone who can listen, be objective, and provide support.

Continue to ask the HCP and staff questions until you understand completely. Rephrase and verbalize what you heard to be sure it is correct. You may want to take a small tape recorder to tape the conversation, but first ask the HCP. Ask how you can learn more. Often the office will have pamphlets or videotapes.

William's comments:

Have the HCP always write out instructions and explain in detail the reasons for recommending new medications and their potential side effects.

Continue to ask the HCP and staff questions until you understand completely.

18. What will we talk about at the first visit?

When you visit your HCP it is crucial to give a concise, organized description of your illness. Avoid long-winded explanations and irrelevant details. Be honest. If you are afraid you have cancer do not say you are "tired and run down" or you are here just for a "checkup." Be prepared on the first visit to give your HCP information for the following five categories:

When you visit your HCP it is crucial to give a concise, organized description of your illness.

1. Chief complaint(s)—what brought you to the HCP today? Express your problem clearly.

2. Present illness—this is where you will tell the story about the chief complaint(s). For example, when did it start? What were your initial symptoms? Try to tell the story in the order from the start to the present time.

3. Past medical history—the HCP will want to know about your health in the past including childhood diseases, hospitalizations, and chronic illnesses.

4. Review of systems—usually in a first complete medical visit the HCP will review symptoms related to different parts of your body.

5. Social history—usually in a first visit the HCP will ask about your occupation, family, stresses, smoking, use of alcohol or illicit drugs, sexual activity.

If you are not honest, life-threatening complications may go undetected by the HCP.

These topics can be very personal, but it is essential to be honest because it can help to determine your illness and treatment. If you are not honest, life-threatening complications may go undetected by the HCP.

19. What should I do about new problems and questions?

Limit new problems to the most important. Written descriptions and your own opinion of the diagnosis will suggest other questions by the provider. Write down the name or diagnosis of the problem and the instructions given by your HCP.

It may also improve your understanding if you ask to have everything explained in lay terms (non-medical terms). Be certain you understand the diagnosis. Laboratory tests, X-rays, or consultations with specialists may be recommended by your HCP for new problems. Do not hesitate to ask how these will confirm the HCP's opinion. Ask if the office has printed information on the new subject to give you and ask what the procedure is to get results of testing and consultations. For example, there may be a special telephone number to call to get results.

20. Will I be given a diagnosis?

After asking more about your complaints, the HCP will probably give you a preliminary diagnosis or an idea of the causes of your illness or symptoms. There may also be a need for an examination as well as laboratory tests, X-rays, or consultations with specialists. If you do not understand something, ask to have it repeated or ask the HCP to draw or write in your notebook. Some practices also provide printed materials relating to a variety of disorders that can help you with understanding your special problem. Ask for any written materials and write down information in your notebook so you will remember what was said and what you are to do when you go home. You must understand information on your illness and all the instructions given to you. Do not rely on memory. If you brought a friend or family member, ask them to take notes on the instructions for you. Before leaving, obtain from one of the office personnel telephone numbers that you can use to get results of tests or to reach the HCP.

Nancy's comments:

I admire HCPs who are honest and clear about advice and your condition.

After asking more about your complaints, the HCP will probably give you a preliminary diagnosis or an idea of the causes of your illness or symptoms.

You must understand information on your illness and all the instructions given to you. Do not rely on memory.

21. Will I be given prescriptions?

The need for prescriptions will be determined by the type of problem and the necessity for early intervention. It is important that you play an active part in improving and maintaining your health. Take any prescriptions and follow treatments as instructed. If you cannot follow the treatment plan (e.g., you cannot take a medication at work), let your HCP know. Do not say you will take medications if you know you will not.

It is important that you play an active part in improving and maintaining your health. Take any prescriptions and follow treatments as instructed.

You should ask about side effects of medications and possible reactions with other drugs you are currently taking (refer to the section on medications). Your HCP or pharmacist may have printed materials on new drugs you will be taking. If you have pills that you stopped taking due to problems, be sure to dispose of them in a safe manner. Never give medications prescribed for you to friends or family to try. Having leftover medications can be a hazard for adults and children. Adults and children can become seriously ill or die from taking leftover or expired medications.

22. Will I receive a treatment plan?

Your HCP or pharmacist may have printed materials on new drugs you will be taking.

You and your HCP should create a treatment plan together. After you and your HCP have developed the treatment plan, follow it closely. Do not say you will follow the treatment plan if you will not (e.g., exercise, low sodium diet). Furthermore, be sure the treatment plan takes into account your lifestyle, religious, and cultural preferences. Make sure you know which follow-up steps to take, when to call and why, and with whom you should speak (e.g., HCP, receptionist, nurse). If you notice problems or side effects, notify your HCP immediately. Some individuals like to make a chart or have a separate calendar so they know what days of the week and time of day to take medications. If you wish to change methods of treatment, then express this to your HCP. You need to be a partner in developing the treatment plan.

23. What is the CBC test that HCPs often order?

A very common laboratory test is called the **complete blood count (CBC)**. This test measures your **red blood cells** (measured by **Hematocrit** and **Hemoglobin**), your **white blood cells (WBC)**, and your **platelets**. The normal values are shown below in **Table 1**. Some primary care HCPs maintain small laboratories and technicians in their offices to draw your CBC. Other HCPs will refer you to a laboratory facility in their building, the local hospital or an independent office.

24. What are some of the other common laboratory tests that might be ordered?

Although the CBC is the most common blood test ordered by primary care HCPs, your HCP may order other laboratory tests based on your symptoms and your examination. These tests appear in **Table 2**.

Table 1 Main Components of Complete Blood Count

Complete Blood Count	Normal Range (Adults)	Clinical Implications If Abnormal
Hematocrit	37–55/100 ml	Anemia, dehydration, shock
Hemoglobin	12–17 gm/dl	Anemia, congestive heart failure, chronic obstructive pulmonary
White blood cells	5,000–10,000/mm3	Infection, diabetes, cancer
Platelets	15,000–450,000/mm3	Trauma, infections, arthritis, cancer, pneumonia

Table 2 Other Common Blood Laboratory Tests

Other Common Values	Normal Range (Adults)	Clinical Implications If Abnormal
Blood sugar (Glucose) fasting	50–110 mg/dl	Diabetes, thyroid, liver problems
Blood Urea Nitrogen (BUN)	10–15 mg/100ml	Kidney disease, dehydration, liver failure, diabetes
Calcium (total)	9.0–10.6 mg/dl	Cancer, thyroid problems, renal failure
Cholesterol	150–250 mg/dl	Heart, liver, or thyroid problems
Creatinine	0.2–0.5 mg/dl	Renal or urinary problems
Magnesium	1.8–3.0 mg/dl	Renal, diabetes, thyroid
Potassium	3.5–5.0 mEq/l	Burns, renal or liver problems
Sodium	132–142 mEq/l	Dehydration, burns, diabetes
Triglycerides	40–150 mg/dl	Thyroid or liver problems

Becky's comments:

I have found that it is so important to carry copies of your blood tests. You can't always assume that your doctor has every copy, especially because the tests aren't always in a centralized location. You can have blood tests at your endocrinologist, primary, gynecologist, and on and on. They are very telling tests, and obtaining a copy of every test will ensure that all of your doctors will have access to the information.

25. Will my HCP want to take a urine sample?

Depending upon your symptoms and your examination, a urine sample may be needed. Usually this can be done at your HCP's office. But if you are having blood drawn at an independent laboratory, you may also have the urine sample collected there. **Table 3** shows some of the common results from a urine sample.

Table 3 Results of Urine Tests

Other Common Values	Normal Range (Adults)	Clinical Implications If Abnormal
Bilrubin	Negative–0.02 mg/dl	Liver disease
Blood in urine	Negative	Renal, burns, malaria
Chloride	110–250 mEq/24 hrs	Dehydration, congestive heart failure
Color	Yellow, straw, amber	Many diseases and infections
Ketone bodies	Negative	Diabetic coma, intestinal problems
Osmolality	Dilute urine < 200 mM, concentrated > 850 mM	Liver, congestive heart failure, high protein or calcium
pH	4.6–8	Urinary tract infections, renal problems, diabetes
Protein (albumin)	Negative or 2–8 mg/dl	Renal, fever, trauma
Sodium	130–200 mEq/24 hrs	Dehydration, renal, diabetes
Specific Gravity	1.003–1.035	Diabetes, renal, water loss
Sugar (glucose)	Negative	Diabetes, heart attack
White Blood Cells	3–4 WBC casts	Bacterial urinary tract infection

26. What routine procedures might be ordered?

Almost all HCPs will want to have the nurse take your weight, blood pressure, pulse, temperature, and respirations before you are put into the examination room. These values can be very helpful in determining what might be wrong with you. For instance, if you have a high fever (normal temperature is 98.6°F), increased blood pressure and increased respirations you may have a respiratory (lung or bronchitis) infection. X-rays may be ordered as routine tests. For example, at an annual physical your HCP may order a chest X-ray. Or an X-ray may be ordered to look for a possible broken bone or sprain.

27. What special procedures might be ordered?

Computed Tomography (CT) Scan—a special X-ray study that takes pictures of the inside of your body. A narrow X-ray beam moves around a section of your body. The images produced are patterned much like slices of bread. These pictures are made to focus on the body part(s) your doctor needs to see.

Magnetic Resonance Imaging (MRI) Scan—this test uses magnetic and low energy radiowaves to produce a series of pictures. It does not use any type of X-ray beam. It is important to tell your HCP of any surgeries or accidents that may have left metal clips or objects in your body.

Ultrasound—is a test that uses sound waves to produce images of organs inside your body. No X-rays or radiation are used in this test.

28. Do I need to tell my HCP if I have a pacemaker or anything metal implanted?

It is very important to tell your HCP on your first visit if you have a pacemaker or anything implanted that is metal (e.g., a pain pump). If you have a pacemaker or certain metal implants you cannot have certain procedures or tests like an MRI performed.

29. Are there special screening tests that my HCP may recommend to prevent cancer?

Usually your primary care HCP will recommend screening tests for cancer according to national guidelines (e.g., the American Cancer Society in the Appendix). Examples of procedures that may be ordered to screen for cancer include:

Colonoscopy—is the examination of the large intestine with a fiberoptic instrument. It allows the physician to look for inflammatory problems, polyps or tumors. This technique allows for specimens to be taken. A baseline colonoscopy is recommended for everyone at age 50 years old to help screen for colorectal cancer.

Mammography—is the use of an X-ray image of the breasts on photographic film to detect cancers that may not be discovered by breast self-exam or the clinical exam of a HCP. Generally, women should have a baseline mammogram at age 40. If there is a family history of breast cancer, you may need a mammogram at an earlier age.

It is very important to tell your HCP on your first visit if you have a pacemaker or anything implanted that is metal.

PART FOUR

Subsequent Visits to Your HCP

What should I take on subsequent visits
to my HCP?

What should I write in my notebook before,
during, and after my appointment?

What should I tell the HCP if I have
a specific symptom?

More . . .

30. What should I take on subsequent visits to my HCP?

On subsequent visits, written notes or reminders are helpful. Write down your questions, progress, and any new problems in your notebook. Be sure to ask if you need refills on medications. Bring all of your medications, vitamins, herbs, and other therapeutic remedies you take in a plastic bag. This will allow the HCP to see everything you are taking at one time. You should discuss unresolved questions, misunderstandings, and new problems. If you have difficulty explaining your problems or understanding your HCP, then take a trusted friend or relative again to assist you. Nursing personnel in your HCP's office can also be helpful.

Nancy's comments:

Take a list of all of your questions and concerns. And be sure to always bring your insurance card!

Write down your questions, progress, and any new problems in your notebook.

Bring all of your medications, vitamins, herbs, and other therapeutic remedies you take in a plastic bag.

31. What should I write in my notebook before, during, and after my appointment?

You can organize a notebook in any way that it will be most helpful for you. You can make sections for: questions before appointments; notes during the appointment; and questions, notes, and symptoms when you are home after the appointment. It is essential that the notebook be helpful for you and your HCP. You may want to think of it as more of a diary of your health and date the page when you write down questions, symptoms, or notes. As will be discussed in the next few questions, it is crucial for you to keep track of ongoing symptoms you have (e.g., pain or fatigue). You can use your notebook to keep a diary of these symptoms.

32. What should I tell the HCP if I have a specific symptom?

If you are communicating with your HCP about a symptom like pain, keep a descriptive record of it. Try to characterize it with words like dull, constant, throbbing, sharp, or burning. When did it start? Have you found something that relieves it? Does it move or radiate to other areas? What makes it worse? Are there associated symptoms, such as fever, dizziness, visual or hearing changes, or weakness? Do you have visible changes (called "signs")? These might be swelling, rash, or bleeding. It is also helpful to rate your symptom on a scale of 0 to 10. For example, with pain 0 = no pain and 10 = worst possible pain. You can also make a chart or table to track your symptom as shown in **Table 4**.

If you have multiple symptoms you may want to chart them on chart the rating on one table as shown in **Table 5**.

33. What questions should I ask or information should I give on a visit to the HCP?

Before arriving at the office you should write any questions down in your notebook. Other specific questions to ask your HCP might include:

1. What did you learn by examining me?
2. What is the cause of my symptom(s)/illness?
3. Should I worry about the symptom(s)/illness?
4. Will you need to do any tests to confirm my diagnosis?
5. How will you treat the symptom(s)/illness?
6. What is my prognosis? What can I expect in the future?

Table 4 Symptom Tracking Chart for Pain

Directions for completing the chart: 1) Rate your pain at each time point on a scale of 0 = no pain to 10 = worst pain, 2) list any medication you have taken at that time and the dosage.

Date	Morning	Mid-Morning	Lunch	Mid-afternoon	Dinner	Bedtime
1/1/2007	Rating = 10 Took 1 vicodin	Rating = 7 No meds	Rating = 8 Took 2 vicodin	Rating = 5 No meds	Rating = 6 Took 1 vicodin	Rating = 8 Took 2 vicodin

Table 5 Chart for Multiple Symptoms

Directions for completing the chart: Rate each symptom on a scale of 0 = no symptom to 10 = worst possible symptom.

Symptom	Day 1	Day 2	Day 3	Day 4	Day 5	Day 6	Day 7
Pain	8	9	6	7	4	3	3
Fatigue	10	8	9	8	10	6	8
Nausea	0	3	1	2	0	1	2

34. How should I phrase any questions I have for the HCP?

It is best to NOT use a leading question that is phrased in such a way that it signals the answers you are hoping for. If you do this you may get an answer that is inaccurate or misleading. It is better to ask who, where, when, how, and why questions. An example of a leading question is: "Have you done a significant number of these operations?" A more effective question would be: "How many of these operations have you done in the last 12 months?"

Continue to ask questions. HCPs are passionate about health care and like to talk about it. Therefore, ask as many questions as you need to.

Continue to ask questions. HCPs are passionate about health care and like to talk about it. Therefore, ask as many questions as you need to. But also remember to thank them. It is rare that HCPs receive words of thanks or gratitude.

35. Do I need to allow my HCP to use me to teach other HCPs?

It is crucial for medical students, nurse practitioner students, and physician assistant students to have clinical experience before graduating and caring for patients on their own. These students will do clinical rotations in the hospital, outpatient and ambulatory facilities, and private offices. You should ALWAYS be asked by your primary HCP or a consultant you are seeing if you are willing to have one or more students examine you. Usually only one student is allowed at a time. You should feel comfortable telling your HCP that you do NOT want a student that day or stating that you NEVER want one. If a student mistakenly enters and starts taking a history, just briefly explain that you would prefer to wait and ONLY see your HCP. Most students are very understanding.

You should ALWAYS be asked by your primary HCP or a consultant you are seeing if you are willing to have one or more students examine you.

36. What do I do if I need a note from the doctor for school or work?

Although with adults many employers trust the individual to be truthful about the need for personal time to see doctors and to try to plan around the office needs, some employers and schools do require notes if you or your family member will be absent due to illness. This is an important topic for you to discuss with your HCP. You need to have reviewed your work or school policy on notes and absences and, if possible, bring a copy to your HCP. However, it is NEVER a guarantee that the HCP will provide you with a note. As your relationship with your HCP develops through subsequent visits and there is a sense of trust, it will be easier. You almost always will have to make a visit to your HCP in order to get a note. Most HCPs will not be able to provide a note if you decide to just take a "sick day" and stay home. You also will need to have new symptoms or an ongoing problem for which you are being evaluated. If you are responsible for taking your child to the pediatrician and you need a note for your child to miss school and you need one to miss work you NEED to be clear with your HCP up front and show them the policies. It is not always possible, but it can be helpful to keep a copy of these notes for yourself in case they ever get lost once you turn them in.

You need to have reviewed your work or school policy on notes and absences and, if possible, bring a copy to your HCP.

37. Do I need to discuss what I want done if my heart stops or I stop breathing?

If you have not already discussed your wishes related to what medical treatments you do or do not want if you become unable to make a decision for yourself, you should discuss this on a subsequent visit. Specifically, you should discuss **advanced directives, healthcare proxies, do not resuscitate orders**, and **living wills**.

An **advanced directive** is a legal document in which you indicate who you want to make medical decisions for you and/or what type of medical treatments you want to receive if you become unable to make decisions for yourself.

A **healthcare proxy** is a person designated in the advanced directive to make healthcare decisions for you if you are not able to. Other terms for this include: healthcare surrogate, a medical proxy and a medical power of attorney.

A **do not resuscitate (DNR)** order is an order placed on your medical chart based on your wishes that you do not want extraordinary life-extending measures to be taken if you stop breathing or your heart stops beating.

A **living will** is a document in which you can state specific instructions regarding your health care, including measures that would prolong your life. You may outline which medical interventions you want to have withheld for a variety of circumstances and which ones you want administered.

Becky's comments:
In a living will, you can also state asset distribution and other things of that nature in addition to healthcare wishes.

PART FIVE

Your Medications

What do I need to tell my HCP about
my medications?

Should I tell my HCP if I have an addiction?

What do I need to know if I receive
a new prescription?

More . . .

38. What do I need to tell my HCP about my medications?

For all medical visits and emergencies, carry a card in your wallet listing all medications and their dosages that you are taking (**Table 6**). Also, list any allergies that you have to medications, bees, or foods, such as peanuts. It is best on first and subsequent visits to try to bring all your prescriptions in their original bottles. This will allow the nurse or HCP to check and make sure you have been given the correct medications and dosages from the pharmacy. It is critical that your HCP always have the most current list of your medications. If your HCP has the most current list they can help make sure you are not on too many medications, or on medications that might cause interactions with other medications, or on medications that may cause side effects for you.

39. Should I tell my HCP if I have an addiction?

It is absolutely vital in an open, honest relationship to tell your HCP of any or all addictions:

- If you have one or more addiction(s)
- What it is (alcohol, smoking, cocaine)
- How long you have had the addiction
- How does the addiction currently affect your health, ability to function, and quality of life?
- Have you tried any methods to stop the addiction in the past? Did these work or not?
- Are you willing to try again to conquer this addiction with the help of your HCP?

Addiction does not mean taking pain medications for legitimate medical reasons. Addiction means taking or

Table 6

Prescription and Dosage	How Much to Take And When?	What Is It For?	Prescribing Physcician	Date Started

using illegal, or legal, substances for pleasure or recreational or social use. Your HCP needs to know this information because the substance you are abusing may seriously affect treatments or medications your HCP may prescribe. Moreover, if you want help for your addiction, your HCP can help you find appropriate resources to help you cope with your addiction.

40. What do I need to know if I receive a new prescription?

If your HCP gives you a new prescription, make sure you can read and understand it.

If your HCP gives you a new prescription, make sure you can read and understand it. Ask important questions and write the responses in your notebook. Some questions may include:

- What is this medicine for?
- How do I take it? (e.g., once a day, three times a day)
- How long do I take it for? (e.g., for 10 days, until it is gone, continuously for months or years)
- What are the side effects? (e.g., nausea or rash)
- What should I do if I have side effects? (e.g., Do I call the HCP's office? Do I go to the hospital?)
- Should I take this medicine on an empty stomach or with food?
- Is it safe to drink alcohol with this medicine?
- Will this medication interfere with any other medications I am taking?
- Are there any other specific instructions I need to know? (e.g., stay out of the sun)
- With newly prescribed medicines: Is it safe to drive?
- Is this medication OK to take with the vitamins or herbs I take?

If these questions are NOT answered by your HCP be sure you discuss any new medications with the pharmacist who fills the prescription so you know exactly what you are taking and why.

41. What if I start the new medication and 2–3 days later I have problems?

Any medication can cause side effects. Many times the side effects may be mild and may be transient (meaning they only last a few days). Yet, it is CRUCIAL that you let your HCP or the nurse know you are having side effects with your new medication. Call your HCP's office in the morning and, if everyone is busy, leave a message for the nurse. If by mid-afternoon you have not heard anything from your HCP's office, call back and talk to the receptionist and hold until the nurse can talk to you. Explain your symptoms and how severe they are. NEVER STOP a medication without talking to your HCP. Some medications need to be slowly tapered off over several days. If your symptoms become severe and you cannot wait to talk to the HCP, call 911 or have a friend or family member drive you to an Urgent Care Center or the Emergency Room.

It is CRUCIAL that you let your HCP or the nurse know you are having side effects with your new medication.

NEVER STOP a medication without talking to your HCP.

42. Is it possible that I might have to live with a minor side effect in order to benefit from a medication?

As stated previously, all medications, vitamins, and herbs can cause side effects. But there are times when the benefits of the medication outweigh a mild side effect. One example is chronic opioid pain medications. Opioids (or narcotics, as many lay people call them) have helped millions of people live with severe pain every day; however, one of the most common side effects is constipation. There are many remedies that patients can use to prevent chronic constipation. In this case most patients with years of chronic pain would prefer to take an opioid medication and have adequate relief so they can enjoy life and deal with potential constipation rather than live with excruciating pain every day.

43. If I am a woman and trying to get pregnant, do I need to worry with new medications?

If you are a woman of childbearing age, you need to let your HCP know if you are trying to have a baby or think you are pregnant. There are many medications that should NOT be given to pregnant women. To be extra cautious, your HCP can order a pregnancy test before you start a new medication.

If you are a woman of childbearing age you need to let your HCP know if you are trying to have a baby or think you are pregnant.

44. Should I be concerned if I take vitamins or herbs and I receive a new medication?

Be sure to remind the HCP and pharmacist if you use any **herbal therapies**, **vitamins**, or **minerals** (e.g., ginseng, licorice, St. John's Wort). These herbal mixtures can have other compounds like common pain relievers mixed in and, when combined with your other medications, they could cause bleeding or other severe complications. Do not start a new vitamin, herb, mineral, or over the counter product (e.g., for cold or flu or sleep) without discussing it with your HCP and/or pharmacist. Do not take vitamins, minerals, or herbs just because a friend or family member recommended them.

45. Will the HCP recommend that I start taking vitamins or herbs?

The use of vitamin supplements used to be controversial. After many years of research, it has been determined that if you are generally healthy and you eat a healthy diet you can meet your nutritional needs through diet alone. However, there are certain individuals of all ages (but especially elderly individuals) who have food allergies or cannot absorb certain foods properly, which can lead to a lack of certain vitamins. Therefore, your HCP may recommend specific vitamin or mineral supplements to ensure that you meet your optimal nutritional needs. Most HCPs would agree that taking a daily multivitamin makes good sense for elderly individuals and those with certain food allergies or dietary restrictions. But ask your HCP first. There are many preparations of multivitamins available and most are not very expensive. Do not start any new supplement without discussing it with your HCP.

46. Is it better to take the original brand or the generic version of the medication?

Ask the HCP or pharmacist if there is a generic version of the drug available and if it is less expensive than the brand name drug. Ask the HCP if an existing medication is comparable to one of the newer ones. Generic versions of a drug should be the same as the original brand name drug, but occasionally patients report they do not feel the generic form works as well as the brand name drug. It is also critical to know that newer medications may cost more (e.g., a newly developed antibiotic) and there may be a comparable medication that costs less. Remember to shop around for the lowest price.

Ask the HCP or pharmacist if there is a generic version of the drug available and if it is less expensive than the brand name drug.

Follow the directions exactly as the HCP has written them. Never stop taking a drug without talking to your HCP. Ask the HCP if the medications being prescribed need to be slowly tapered off.

47. What if my HCP only gives me samples of a medication?

It is important for you to take the sample exactly as the HCP prescribes. You may want them to write it down because instructions may not be on the sample.

Tell the staff exactly what the side effects are. Do NOT stop the medication until you hear from your HCP.

There are many different medications on the market in each category of medicine (like different antibiotics, different cardiac medicines, and different pain medications). Most medical offices have some samples of the many different medications they prescribe. It is often difficult to know which one medication will work best for you. Rather than having you buy a 30-day supply of a medication and have it not work or cause side effects, the HCP may want to give you a sample. It is important for you to take the sample exactly as the HCP prescribes. You may want them to write it down because instructions may not be on the sample. Before the sample medication runs out (at least 2–3 days), it is your responsibility to call your HCP's office. Let the staff know if the medication is helping. If it is helping and you feel better, give the staff the name and phone number of the pharmacy where you would like the prescription to be called in. If it is NOT helping you, let the staff know that as well. The HCP will then decide whether to have you come back for a visit or prescribe another medication. If at ANY time you are having side effects from the medication, immediately call your HCP's office. Tell the staff exactly what the side effects are. Do NOT stop the medication until you hear from your HCP. Some medications require that you wean off them slowly.

PART SIX

Contacting Your HCP's Office by Telephone

What should I do if I need to call my HCP's office during office hours?

What is a good time of day to call my HCP's office?

What if I want my test results?

More . . .

48. What should I do if I need to call my HCP's office during office hours?

Before calling the office, organize your thoughts and questions. What is the problem or question you are calling about? When did it begin? Is this an urgent matter or can the reply wait 24–48 hours? Have a pad and pencil handy to write down any instructions that you are given.

If your problem is urgent or an emergency, call your HCP's office early in the workday. If your problem is routine and can wait then call in during mid-day or the afternoon.

49. What is a good time of day to call my HCP's office?

If your problem is urgent or an emergency, call your HCP's office early in the workday. If your problem is routine and can wait then call in during mid-day or the afternoon. Be sure to ask how your HCP would like to be contacted—telephone or email. If your HCP would like you to call, ask for the phone number and if there is an extension. The HCP and staff will triage calls and they must deal with the most urgent ones first. If you call the office and leave a message and your problem becomes an emergency, do not hesitate to call 911 or have a family member or friend take you to an urgent care center or an emergency room at a hospital. Do not go to your HCP's office because they will not have the equipment that an urgent care center or emergency room will have.

Many offices will tell you that if they do NOT call you then you may assume your test results are normal. Do NOT settle for this. You have the right to know all your test results even if they are normal.

50. What if I want my test results?

Many offices will tell you that if they do NOT call you then you may assume your test results are normal. Do NOT settle for this. You have the right to know all your test results even if they are normal. Call your HCP's office 1–3 days after the results should be in to ask about the results. Write down the results or request that they mail you a copy. Make sure they explain everything to your satisfaction. If you request copies, you may want to keep a file of laboratory results and results of procedures like MRIs and CT scans.

51. What if I only speak with the receptionist or nurse?

It is difficult for the HCP to take every telephone call. Frequently, the question you may have can be answered by other office staff such as the receptionist, nurse or billing clerk. Or the staff member may be able to ask the HCP the question in between patients and call you back with the answer. However, if your question is still NOT answered adequately and you would like to talk to your HCP, leave a message requesting that they return your call and why. You may have to wait 24–48 hours for the HCP to return your call.

If your question is still NOT answered adequately and you would like to talk to your HCP, leave a message requesting that they return your call and why.

52. What should I do if I need a refill on my medication?

Today, many pharmacies will call or fax your HCP's office for you to get a refill on your medication. This saves time for both you and your HCP, but some offices prefer that you call and leave a message asking for your refill. If your HCP likes you to call and leave a message for refills on your medication, be sure to have the bottle in front of you. Leave your name, date of birth, telephone number (in case there are problems), the name of the medication, the dosage, and how you are taking it. Also leave the name and phone number of your pharmacy (this often is on your medication bottle). Be sure to state in the message if you are having any problems with the medication. Call for any refills at least 2–3 days before you will need the medication.

If your HCP likes you to call and leave a message for refills on your medication, be sure to have the bottle in front of you.

53. *What should I do if I need to reach my HCP on weekends or after office hours?*

If your problem is truly an emergency you should NOT wait to call your HCP. Call 911 or have someone take you to the Emergency Department of your local hospital.

If your problem is truly an emergency you should NOT wait to call your HCP. Call 911 or have someone take you to the Emergency Department of your local hospital. If your problem is not a life-threatening emergency but cannot wait until the next business day, then you have several choices. Today there are many "Urgent Care Centers" in most communities. One may be associated with your HCP or your insurance carrier. These centers tend to be open in the evenings and on weekends. You may choose to go to an Urgent Care Center. Unless you visit this center frequently, they will not know your history. Thus, you may prefer to call your HCP's answering service. All HCPs have someone "on call" to talk to patients who have urgent needs that cannot wait until the next business day. Before you need this service (like when you first select your HCP) you should ask what phone number to call for "after hours or on call" care. Sometimes it is the same as the routine office number. Other times the HCP may use a completely different number for the answering service. Generally, a telephone operator (who is NOT a medical person) will answer the call). Briefly explain why you need to talk to the HCP on call and be sure to give them your name, birth date, and phone number. Do NOT give too much detail because the operator is not a trained medical person. Once you have left a message, be sure to STAY OFF your phone so that the HCP can call you back.

Once you have left a message, be sure to STAY OFF your phone so that the HCP can call you back.

PART SEVEN

Consultants or Specialists and Second Opinions

What are consultants or specialists?

How do I get to see a consultant?

What are subspecialists?

More . . .

54. What are consultants or specialists?

Consultants (or specialists) are healthcare providers other than your primary HCP who are asked to give an opinion about your condition. Sometimes a consultation is performed because your physician would like the advice and counsel of another physician. Consultants or specialists in the field of medical care have multiplied along with new means for diagnosis and treatment. These specialists play a valuable advisory and support role for general healthcare providers.

55. How do I get to see a consultant?

Your HCP will make a referral to a consultant who is specially trained in the area of concern.

Your HCP will make a referral to a consultant who is specially trained in the area of concern. For example, it might be a **Cardiologist** for a heart or blood pressure issue, or an **Urologist** for problems or diseases of the urinary tract, bladder or kidneys, or a **Neurologist** for problems or diseases of the nervous system, or an **Oncologist** for treating cancer. **Surgical Oncologists** specialize in cancer surgery; **Medical Oncologists** specialize in treatment with chemotherapy, hormonal therapy, and biologic therapy; and **Radiation Oncologists** specialize in treating with radiation.

The nurse or receptionist may make an appointment for you with the consultant or the consultant's office may call you to set up the appointment. Lastly, your HCP may prefer to send a written consultation request. If you have a busy schedule you may want to call and make the appointment with the consultant after your HCP has sent the request for the consultation.

56. *What are subspecialists?*

Today there are specialists—like a **general surgeon** who performs operations of many different types. But, there are also subspecialists in surgery. A **colorectal surgeon** will perform surgery on the intestinal tract, colon, rectum and organs affected by the intestine. A **vascular surgeon** performs surgery on disorders of the blood vessels. **Neurosurgeons** specialize in surgery of the brain, brain stem, skull, spine, spinal cord and nerves. There are also **pediatric surgeons** who operate on children from newborns to teenagers. Your HCP will help you find the appropriate subspecialist if you or your family need one.

57. *What questions should I ask the consultant?*

We will use the example of being sent to a surgeon for consultation. You may adapt these questions to ask a consultant based on the type of specialist or subspecialist you are visiting.

Questions might include the following:

- Why do I need surgery?
- Will you explain exactly what type of surgery you suggest?
- Are there less invasive treatments than surgery?
- What will happen if I decide to postpone this surgery for awhile?
- What will happen if I decide NOT to have surgery?
- What are the benefits of this surgery?
- What are the potential complications of surgery and how serious are they?

Your HCP will help you find the appropriate subspecialist if you or your family need one.

You may adapt these questions to ask a consultant based on the type of specialist or subspecialist you are visiting.

- How many of these procedures have you performed?
- How long will I need to stay in the hospital and/or home?
- What can I expect during the recovery period?
- If I were your family member (daughter, mother, etc.) would you recommend this surgery?
- What hospital or facility will you use?
- Will my insurance cover this completely or will I have to pay something?
- What is your philosophy about pain management?

58. Will I hear about the consultation and what should I do in the meantime?

Once you have seen the consultant, a timely report should be sent to your primary HCP. Your HCP should contact you and report the recommendations of the consultant.

Once you have seen the consultant, a timely report should be sent to your primary HCP. Your HCP should contact you and report the recommendations of the consultant. Be sure you understand the diagnosis and treatment that the consultant is recommending. Make a follow-up appointment with the consultant if needed to clarify how long you need to follow the regimen including medications and other instructions.

In order to take responsibility for your health and well-being you should also review the results of tests and reports from the consultants with your HCP so that you understand everything. Your HCP should help you monitor whether you need to continue to see the specialist regularly or not.

59. What should I do if I want a second opinion?

If you are unsure about what your HCP or consultant recommends, you may want to get advice from another HCP or specialist. This is called a second opinion. This involves having your medical records reviewed by another HCP in the same specialty to see what treatment they would recommend. Most insurance providers will cover the cost of a second opinion. Your original primary HCP or consultant should NOT be offended if you ask for a second opinion. If you decide you want a second opinion you may ask your HCP to suggest the names of other qualified HCPs or consultants. If you decided to have a second opinion, be clear about the purpose of the visit when you make the appointment. Make sure all copies of your laboratory and test results are sent or carry them with you. Also be sure that any recommendations that you receive during the second opinion are sent back to your primary HCP.

If you decided to have a second opinion, be clear about the purpose of the visit when you make the appointment.

60. What records should I take for a second opinion or a consultant?

Your HCP should send a letter or fax ahead to give the consultant or secondary HCP some of your past medical history and explain the purpose for the referral. Yet, it is still helpful if you take any current copies of reports from laboratory tests, X-rays, MRIs, CT scans or other procedures with you. This is one reason it is helpful to have a file at home with all of your test results. If you can take some of these reports or be sure they are sent it can save time and help prevent having to repeat the same test twice for different providers. Also take a current list of all of your medications or carry all of the bottles in a plastic bag.

It is still helpful if you take any current copies of reports from laboratory tests, X-rays, MRIs, CT scans or other procedures with you.

PART EIGHT

Pediatric HCPs for Children

Do I need a separate pediatric HCP for my children?

Do I need to have my children immunized?

What type of records do I need to keep
for my children?

More . . .

61. Do I need a separate pediatric HCP for my children?

From birth until about 16–18 years old, it is often best to have your children seen by a Pediatrician or NP or PA who specializes in pediatrics. This will be the primary care HCP for your child/children. Once they reach adulthood they will want to see an internist unless your entire family is seen by a Family HCP.

62. Do I need to have my children immunized?

Immunizations have had a far greater impact on health in the developed nations than all of the other health services put together. Only a few decades ago smallpox, cholera, paralytic polio, diphtheria, whooping cough, and tetanus killed large numbers of people. These diseases have been controlled successfully by immunization in the United States and other developed countries. Unfortunately, many Americans have been lax about getting childhood immunizations, so there has been an increase in measles, mumps, and rubella. Work with your child's HCP to be sure they receive all the appropriate immunizations. **Table 7** shows the recommended schedule.

63. What type of records do I need to keep for my children?

It is very important to have accurate records of any serious illnesses and vaccinations (check to be sure which vaccinations are essential) for each child. If you move from town to town or change your primary HCP, be sure to provide these records to your new HCP for each child. Keep a copy of your children's records in a safe

Table 7 Recommended Immunization Schedule

Age	Immunization
Newborn	Hepatitis B (or later as directed by HCP)
2 months	DPT , Hep B, HIB , Rota, PCV, IPV
4 months	DPT, HIB, Rota, PCV, IPV
6 months	DPT, HIB, Rota, PCV, yearly influenza
12–15 months	DPT, Hep B, HIB,PCV, IPV, Measles, Mumps (MMR), Rubella, Varicella, Hep A (2 doses)
18 months	DPT, Hep B, IPV, yearly influenza
4–6 years	DTAP, IPV, MMR, Varicella

DPT (diphtheria, pertussis, tetanus), IPV (inactivate polio virus) and HIB (hemophilus influenza B), Rota (rotavirus), Hep B (hepatitis B), Hep A (hepatitis A), PCV (pneumococcal)

place. Once your children go to college or are on their own, provide them a list of vaccinations, childhood illnesses (e.g., measles, mumps, and rubella) and the years. Also tell them if they did NOT have certain childhood diseases—especially rubella (German Measles) for females because this can be dangerous to have when they are pregnant later in life.

64. What should I tell the HCP when my child is ill?

When a child is sick and he/she cannot tell you or the primary HCP what is wrong, it is essential for you to explain how the child is acting differently than normal. For example, the child may not be eating, may be less active, pulling at one or both ears, or crying constantly. Describe what is disturbing to you as a parent, especially

When a child is sick and he/she cannot tell you or the primary HCP what is wrong, it is essential for you to explain how the child is acting differently than normal.

for children who cannot verbalize. Also, be sure to report anything teachers mention as change (e.g., a lack of attention, moving closer to the board, inability to stay awake).

PART NINE

Health Care for the Elderly

At what age is an individual considered elderly?

Will my primary care HCP know how to treat conditions I may develop when I am 65 years and older?

What is the difference between gerontology and geriatrics?

More . . .

65. At what age is an individual considered elderly?

People age at different rates so it is hard to define what ages make people "elderly." Old age consists of ages nearing the average lifespan of human beings, and thus, the end of the human life cycle. Although a person 55 years of age or older is defined as elderly by the New York State Human Rights Law, the majority of definitions of elderly currently refer to individuals who are equal to or greater than 65 years old. Some actually define "early elderly" as 65–74 years old and "old elderly" as anyone over 75 years old. For this book we will consider elderly to be 65 years old or greater.

66. Will my primary care HCP know how to treat conditions I may develop when I am 65 years and older?

As explained in the beginning, once you or your HCP consider you elderly—or at about 65 years or older—you may want to switch from your primary HCP to a **Geriatrician** or NP or PA who specializes in geriatrics (care of the elderly). As medical science has advanced and individuals are living longer, we have learned that there are certainly some unique and specific health issues that may occur as we become elderly. As one patient said to us a number of years ago—"It is not the Golden Years, it is the Rusty Years."

Once you or your HCP consider you elderly—or at about 65 years or older—you may want to switch from your primary HCP to a Geriatrician or NP or PA who specializes in geriatrics (care of the elderly).

67. What is the difference between gerontology and geriatrics?

Gerontology is the scientific study of old age. **Geriatrics** is the discipline of medicine that focuses on prevention, diagnosis, treatment and long-term care in older adults. That is why you want to have a HCP who specializes in Geriatrics.

68. What is involved in a comprehensive geriatric physical examination?

This is an evaluation for an elderly patient (> 65 years old). A Comprehensive Geriatric Physical Examination focuses on the physical health, mental health, functional status, social well-being, and spiritual well-being. As we get older we all develop ailments as the organs in our body no longer function as well as they used to. The goal is to complete a thorough and comprehensive examination and then develop a plan of care that will maximize independence and prevent disability. It is especially helpful to have a comprehensive geriatric physical examination if you retire in your 60s and decide to relocate to another state or country. This would allow your new HCP to do a comprehensive and thorough physical examination.

A Comprehensive Geriatric Physical Examination focuses on the physical health, mental health, functional status, social well-being, and spiritual well-being.

69. What activities can I continue to do while maintaining my health as I pass 65 years old?

Unless your HCP has given you any restrictions, if you feel well and enjoy some part-time or full-time work you may continue to do so. There are individuals who continue to work into their 80s and 90s. If you have health limitations or if there are activities like traveling that you want to pursue, you may want to retire in your 60s or 70s.

In general, for physical and mental health it is advisable to keep active when you are over 65 years.

In general, for physical and mental health it is advisable to keep active when you are over 65 years. You may want to travel or become involved in community volunteer work. It is important to continue to eat nutritious meals and get some exercise (e.g., walking or water exercises).

70. What if I feel overwhelmed by taking care of myself, my spouse, and our house?

Many individuals find it tedious to continue to prepare meals and care for a house and yard. There are many nice "retirement communities" available with minimal to maximum services. There are also "life care" communities. These communities allow you to enter while you are mobile (e.g., live in an apartment or condominium) and as you or your spouse need more services you can have them brought to your apartment or slowly transition into the long-term full-care option. The idea is to provide you with care until you pass away. There are also nursing homes that are long-term care institutions with inpatient beds, and which offer around-the-clock nursing care, as well as medical, social, and personal services. Usually your HCP may know of different retirement, life care communities, and nursing homes in your area. You need to plan early because some will not accept you if you are over 80 years old, or if you are not able to ambulate (get around without a wheelchair or walker) on your own without help when you first enter. Additionally, some have long waiting lists.

Usually your HCP may know of different retirement, life care communities, and nursing homes in your area.

71. How can my HCP help if I have trouble caring for myself but do not want to leave my home?

As you grow older you have many choices of how to take care of your medical ailments and where to live. Your HCP can help discuss these with you. In addition to considering a retirement center or life care arrangement you may opt to stay at home and have home health services. There are many excellent home healthcare agencies. These agencies provide a broad range of health and social services in your home (like a nurse to help with medications or a physical therapist to help with exercises so that you do not fall). Your HCP or a social worker can help you decide if home health care is your best option. You can obtain additional information about home health care through the American Academy of Home Care Physicians at *www.aahcp.org/aahcp* or by calling 410-676-7966.

In addition to considering a retirement center or life care arrangement you may opt to stay at home and have home health services.

Your HCP or a social worker can help you decide if home health care is your best option.

72. If I decide on home health care, will my insurance cover the cost?

Depending on your medical condition and whether you have Medicare and supplemental insurance, the costs for some or all of your home health services (e.g., visits by a nurse, a home health aide, or homemaker) should be paid for. If you have purchased a long-term care policy this may cover additional costs like medical equipment, 24-hour care by an aide and other items required for your care.

If you are over 55 and in good health, you may want to consider buying a long-term care insurance policy that will cover services in your home or in a nursing home. It is better to purchase these policies when you are younger and in better health.

73. Now that I am elderly I find I am developing new problems and my body organs seem to be slowing down. Is there anything the HCP can do for me?

Many medications and treatments are now available for many conditions unique to elderly patients and significant research is being conducted to find additional treatments. Depending on the problem, your HCP may need to schedule laboratory tests or imaging studies, or have you see a consultant. Your treatment will depend on the health issue the HCP discovers.

Forgetfulness, or cognitive impairment, is one of the more common problems for the elderly. Thus, it is even more important that you have a notebook and write down everything you are told. Be sure you understand the problem and the treatment in lay terms. Ask the nurses for written or printed information about your condition or treatment to take home.

Becky's comments:

As you get older, it might be a good idea to have a family member or close friend go to appointments with you. It helps to have someone there with you to remember all of the questions you may have for your healthcare provider, as well as another pair of ears and memory to catch everything that you will learn or hear during the appointment.

74. What if part of my problem is keeping track of my medications?

Another problem for many elderly is keeping track of medications. This may be partly due to forgetfulness, but it can also be due to the number of medications the individual has to take every day. Go over your medications with your HCP and see if any can be discontinued or scheduled at an easier time like bedtime. Ask a nurse in your HCP's office to help you plan a calendar so you know what to take at different times of each day (e.g., before breakfast, with breakfast, with lunch, midafternoon, dinner time, bedtime). It is also extremely helpful to buy a pillbox at the drug store that has slots for four times a day and for seven days of the week. If you sit down and put all the pills for one week in the box (or have a spouse, friend or caretaker do so), you can double check whether you have taken pills on a specific day or time of day. If you open that time slot and the pills are gone, you took them. If they are still there you may have forgotten and need to take them right away. Be sure you clarify with your HCP on each medication what to do if you miss a dose. For example, for some medications if it is late two hours or more you should NOT take them, while for other medications it is important to take the medication even if it is late.

It is also extremely helpful to buy a pillbox at the drug store that has slots for four times a day and for seven days of the week.

Be sure you clarify with your HCP on each medication what to do if you miss a dose.

75. *What are my options if I am elderly and terminally ill?*

As discussed in Part 4, question 34, it is helpful to plan for serious illness before it happens. You should consider an advanced directive, living will, and do not resuscitate order. Whether you have planned for this or not, if you are terminally ill, your HCP should help you consider your options and help you make the decision that is best for you and your family. If you are terminally ill and there are no other medical treatments that may help you, then you may want to consider Hospice. **Hospice** is a philosophy of care that helps you live the rest of your life with quality and dignity and to be symptom-free when your life expectancy is six months or less. Hospices provide volunteer support, pastoral, and social work care. Providers from hospice apply the principles of palliative care. These principles are generally focused on relief of symptoms and attention to each individual patient's spiritual, emotional, and physical concerns (quality of life) rather than resolving specific illness episodes.

Hospice care can be provided in your home, in the hospital, in a nursing home, or in a private hospice house. Medicare will cover the cost of hospice and provide you with any medical equipment, your medications, and support by an interdisciplinary team (nurse, aide, social worker, chaplain, and more). They will communicate directly with your HCP so you and your family do not need to worry.

76. Should I tell my HCP if I am being abused?

It is critical for you to tell at least your HCP if you are being abused. Individuals can be abused at any age, especially when you are 65 years or older. This is called **elder abuse** and there are several types. **Physical abuse** is the infliction of bodily injury and may be manifested by lacerations, fractures, soft tissue trauma, burns, or bruises. **Sexual abuse** is any form of intimate sexual activity without consent. **Emotional** or **psychological abuse** is the infliction of mental anguish, such as intimidation by yelling, insulting, threatening, or silence. **Financial exploitation** is the misuse of another person's funds or assets without his or her explicit knowledge or consent. **Caregiver neglect** is the malicious neglect by a caregiver of an older person's needs, whether for retaliation, disinterest, or financial incentives.

It is critical for you to tell at least your HCP if you are being abused. Individuals can be abused at any age, especially when you are 65 years or older.

PART TEN

Treatment Options

What do I need to know about my treatment options?

Will I need to be involved in a clinical trial or research to get treatment?

What is informed consent associated with clinical trials and research?

More . . .

77. *What do I need to know about my treatment options?*

Ask your HCP about any suggested treatments. Be sure you discuss all possible treatments and you are a partner in the decision making. Ask if there are multiple options for treatment or only one. If you do not understand the explanations or information be sure to have it repeated. Ask for written materials or for your HCP to draw things for you. You may want to repeat information back to the HCP to be sure you understood correctly. Make notes in your notebook. Be sure that any and all treatment options take into account any cultural, religious, dietary, or ethnic preferences. Do not assume that your HCP knows what holidays or religious or dietary restrictions by which you abide.

78. *Will I need to be involved in a clinical trial or research to get treatment?*

No patient is required to participate in clinical trials or research studies. **Clinical trials** are research studies to test the effectiveness of new treatments on human beings. Some clinical trials or research studies are designed to test treatments for specific medical problems like cancer or diabetes; however, some are designed to test treatments for symptoms like pain or nausea. Your HCP or a consultant may recommend a particular clinical trial or research study. Be sure the research is fully explained to you and remember that it is *voluntary*. If you agree to take part in a study and later decide you want to withdraw, you may do that. If you would like to find out more information regarding clinical trials you can contact the National Institutes of Health (Appendix), or Centerwatch (Appendix). If you want information specifically related to clinical trials for cancer, you may contact the National Cancer Institute (Appendix).

79. What is informed consent associated with clinical trials and research?

Certain research is essential to help discover new treatments and medications. But, you MUST be sure you want to volunteer. If you agree to be in a study you must be fully informed. This is called **informed consent**. This means that you understand and give permission for a treatment, procedure, or medication even though there may be benefits and complications.

If you agree to be in a study you must be fully informed.

There are 3 major steps to informed consent:

1. The procedure, treatment, or medication and any risks should be explained to you in lay terms that you can understand. This explanation may not be given while you are sleepy or sedated.

2. Anything you do NOT understand MUST be explained to you in such a way that you thoroughly understand what is being said.

3. You and the individual explaining the procedure, treatment, or medication must both sign a consent form. Additionally, a witness should sign. The witness may be another health care provider or a family member or friend.

80. Are there specific questions I should ask about clinical trials?

You may develop a list of questions to ask about a clinical trial that is being offered to you. Any questions should be written in your notebook so you do not forget.

Examples of questions you might ask are listed below:

- Is there a clinical trial for which I would be eligible?
- What is the purpose of the study?
- What kinds of tests and treatments does the study involve?
- What does this treatment do?
- Will I know which treatment I receive?
- What is likely to happen in my case with, or without, this new treatment?
- What are my other choices and their advantages and disadvantages?
- How could the study affect my daily life?
- What side effects can I expect from the study? Can the side effects be controlled?
- Will I have to be hospitalized? If so, how often and for how long?
- Will the study cost me anything? Will any of the treatment be free?
- If I am harmed as a result of the research, what treatment would I be entitled to?
- What type of long-term follow-up care is part of the study?
- Has the treatment been used to treat other types of diseases?

81. Will there be things I can do at home for myself?

Ask what you can do to help yourself. For example, you may need to increase your exercise, decrease your sodium intake, or implement other self-care activities. It is important that you do as much to help yourself as possible. Continue as many daily activities, hobbies, and sports as possible. Maintain social contacts.

82. If I am having an ongoing treatment, how will I receive feedback on the effectiveness of the treatment?

It is your health and your treatment. It is important for you to know how the treatment is progressing and whether it is effectively treating your condition. There are several ways to obtain this information. Before you start treatment you should discuss with your HCP or specialist (whoever is prescribing the treatment) how and when to discuss your progress on treatment. Several options include:

Before you start treatment you should discuss with your HCP or specialist (whoever is prescribing the treatment) how and when to discuss your progress on treatment.

1. Your HCP might send you a letter updating your progress at specified intervals, such as every 3 months.

2. Another is to have scheduled telephone calls about your progress every 3 months.

3. Lastly, it may be more beneficial for you to schedule an appointment with your HCP on a regular basis like every 3 months. This can be most helpful because it gives you more time to ask questions and the HCP can schedule laboratory tests to monitor your treatment at the same time.

83. Are there complementary therapies that I can use with the treatment ordered by my HCP?

According to most complementary practitioners, the purpose of treatment is to restore balance and facilitate the body's own healing responses rather than to target individual disease processes or use medications to stop troublesome symptoms.

It is important to understand that this holistic approach is not unique to complementary practice. Your primary HCP, for example, should follow similar principles.

Complementary and alternative medicine (CAM) refers to healing treatment(s) used together with mainstream, hospital-based medical practice. There are a wide variety of approaches to improve health and treat symptoms. According to most complementary practitioners, the purpose of treatment is to restore balance and facilitate the body's own healing responses rather than to target individual disease processes or use medications to stop troublesome symptoms. The philosophical base underlying the use of many complementary therapies differs from the conventional Western medical model. While medicine seeks to eliminate, correct, or cure the underlying problem, the purpose for using CAM in other systems of health care is to achieve harmony and balance in the person. Practitioners of CAM may use a package of care, which could include modification of lifestyle, dietary change, and exercise as well as a specific treatment. Thus, a medical herbalist may give counseling, an exercise regimen, guidance on breathing and relaxation, dietary advice, and an herbal prescription. It is important to understand that this holistic approach is not unique to complementary practice. Your primary HCP, for example, should follow similar principles.

The term complementary has been preferred, because it conveys that these therapies are used in conjunction with, rather than as replacement for, medical treatment. The term alternative therapy conveys that a therapy is used in place of a medical treatment.

You should discuss with your HCP if you wish to use complementary therapies. Many HCPs will refer you to appropriate licensed therapists.

Common complementary therapies include the following:
- Acupressure or Acupuncture
- Aqua therapy (therapy in a pool)
- Chiropractic therapy
- Healing Touch
- Herbal therapy
- Homoeopathy
- Hypnosis
- Massage therapy
- Meditation
- Nutritional therapy
- Reiki
- Relaxation therapy
- Yoga

84. What do I do if I have questions after I go home?

Ask your HCP for the best way to follow up if you have questions after your visit. Should you call the office and leave a message with the nurse or receptionist for non-urgent questions? Ask what hours you can contact the office. Many offices close during lunch time. HCPs need a little break each day, so they often ask that you call before or after lunch time. Usually you can expect an answer within 24–48 hours for non-urgent replies. Also, ask for the procedure if the problem is urgent (e.g., call your HCP's office or call 911 or go to the emergency room).

PART ELEVEN

Financial Concerns

What if I have questions about my insurance?

What is Medicare insurance?

How do I know if I am eligible for Medicare?

More . . .

85. What if I have questions about my insurance?

If you have insurance and you are going to see your primary HCP or a consultant for the first time, you should make sure they accept your insurance and you understand what your portion (co-pay) will be.

If you have insurance and you are going to see your primary HCP or a consultant for the first time, you should make sure they accept your insurance and you understand what your portion (co-pay) will be. Often the person making your appointment or a billing clerk can answer this question. Additionally, if you receive a bill that you believe is incorrect you should call the HCP's office and discuss the bill with the billing clerk. Sometimes mistakes are made, or your insurance may not have covered as much of the visit as expected. If the issue regarding your bill has to do with your insurance company then you will want to call that company. The phone number for questions on your insurance is usually listed on the front or back of your insurance card. Medical bills can be confusing to read and understand so it may be helpful to take the bill to your HCP's office and ask the billing clerk to review and explain it to you.

86. What is Medicare insurance?

Medicare is a federally funded health insurance program implemented in 1966 by President Lyndon Johnson under his Great Society Act as a health insurance program for the elderly. Medicare has two parts. Part A is considered the hospital insurance and helps cover inpatient care in the hospital, skilled nursing care, and some home health care as well as hospice care. Part B is the part that covers your HCP services, diagnostic tests, laboratory tests, and medical equipment.

87. How do I know if I am eligible for Medicare?

In general, if you are 65 years or older and you (or your spouse) have paid Medicare taxes through your paychecks for at least 10 years, you are eligible for Part A of Medicare. You automatically become eligible for Part B if you are eligible for Part A. Part B is voluntary, so you must be sure to request the information, review it carefully, and enroll. If you are not enrolled for Medicare you can obtain the information by calling 1-800-772-1213 or 1-800-633-4227, or it is available on the Internet at *www.medicare.gov*. If you need additional coverage to help you with co-payments you may want to buy Medigap. **Medigap** is a form of private supplementary insurance. The link on the Internet at the Medicare website: *www.Medicare.gov/MGcompare/home*.asp can help you find choices of private agencies that offer Medigap in your area. Pick the one that best meets your needs. You may prefer to enroll in a Medicare HMO (Medicare managed care), which is a medical plan under Medicare. A Medicare HMO can offer you additional benefits, but it might limit you to specific hospitals or doctors. Be sure to ask if your HCP accepts Medicare and your form of Medigap or the Medicare HMO.

If you need additional coverage to help you with co-payments you may want to buy Medigap.

You may prefer to enroll in a Medicare HMO (Medicare managed care), which is a medical plan under Medicare.

88. Will my HCP accept my medicare insurance?

It is voluntary for your HCP to be a Medicare provider. They must enroll to be a provider; however, most primary care HCPs and Geriatricians accept Medicare Part B insurance. But, remember, just as your HCP has to enroll to be a provider, you must enroll to have Part B of the Medicare Insurance. It is important to call ahead

It is voluntary for your HCP to be a Medicare provider. They must enroll to be a provider; however, most primary care HCPs and Geriatricians accept Medicare Part B insurance.

and ask the billing clerk if they accept Medicare and any other supplemental insurance you may have (e.g., Blue Cross Blue Shield, Aetna). If they do not accept your insurance they may be able to refer you to a qualified HCP who does accept Medicare.

89. What is Medicaid insurance?

Medicaid is a joint federal and state program that provides health insurance to individuals who have low incomes and limited savings. Medicaid was enacted in 1964 as part of the federal and state welfare system. Before Medicaid was started physicians and hospitals often gave charity care or billed on a sliding scale (meaning individuals would pay what they could).

90. Will my HCP accept Medicaid insurance?

With Medicaid your HCP has to volunteer to be a provider, just as with Medicare; however, most primary care HCPs do accept Medicaid. In order to be sure your visits, tests, and medications are covered, it is best to call your HCP's office and ask the billing clerk if they accept Medicaid. If they do not accept Medicaid they usually can refer you to another HCP who will accept your insurance.

91. What if I am worried about how much office visits, medications, procedures or treatments will cost?

Ask your HCP or any of the staff about charges at your first visit or any other visit. Many individuals are afraid to ask their HCPs about fees. If you do not ask, then you may be worrying about this important detail when your HCP is describing a test or other important health information to you. If you discuss charges up front it will make you less anxious and allow the HCP and staff to know if you are financially strapped. If that is the case, your HCP can possibly give you medication samples, write prescriptions for generic drugs, and set up a reasonable payment plan for you.

PART TWELVE

The Use of Computers in Medical Care

Why is there a computer in my HCP's
examination room?

What if my HCP is typing away and it bothers me?

How can I use a computer to collect information
on my health?

More . . .

92. Why is there a computer in my HCP's examination room?

Most offices and many hospitals now have electronic medical records. This means that your HCP enters all of the important information from your visit and phone calls into the computer. This will include operating reports, lab results, and much more. This allows the HCP and other office staff to look up your medications and other health information quickly rather than searching and searching for your chart.

93. What if my HCP is typing away and it bothers me?

Although it does often save the HCP time to type your answers into the computer while you are talking, it is important for you to speak up and let the HCP know you would rather they face you and make eye contact rather than typing while you are talking. They can type in the information later after you have left the office. They may request to make a few notes on a piece of paper during your visit so they will remember what to enter into the computer later.

94. How can I use a computer to collect information on my health?

If you have a computer and internet access at home, it is very easy today to find information regarding any type of medical problem. But, YOU MUST BE CAREFUL. There are many internet sites that are NOT maintained by medical professionals. Be sure you are getting information from a credible medical or health website. We have listed many in the Appendix of this book. For example, websites sponsored by healthcare foundations or associations such as the American Cancer Society or the American Diabetes Association are credible websites. AVOID sites done by one individual with your same health problem. This individual's experience may be very different than yours.

95. What if I do not own a computer or have access to the internet?

There are different places you can go to use computers and many of them are free. The first place to consider is your local Public Library. Libraries often have a collection of computers with Internet access and the librarians can help you find the information you want. There are also places called "Internet Cafes." These are usually coffee shops or restaurants that have some computers for use while you have something to drink or eat. You also may have a family member or friend who will allow you to use their computer. Lastly, you can often sign up for inexpensive computer classes at libraries or other community centers and then use the computer for free after or before class.

If you have a computer and internet access at home, it is very easy today to find information regarding any type of medical problem.

Libraries often have a collection of computers with Internet access and the librarians can help you find the information you want.

PART THIRTEEN

Quality of Life Issues

What should I say if I want to talk to the physician about things that are not physical?

If I have ongoing health problems and I am feeling anxious or down should I tell my HCP?

Should I tell my HCP if my illness is affecting my social life?

More . . .

96. What should I say if I want to talk to the physician about things that are not physical?

If you are honest and discuss physical, psychological, social, and spiritual issues, then all decisions about your health will be made while taking into account what will positively increase your quality of life.

When individuals are sick, especially if it is a chronic illness, it affects them physically, psychologically, socially, and spiritually. We like to refer to this as Quality of Life (**physical well-being**, **psychological well-being**, **social well-being**, and **spiritual well-being**). These topics are often difficult to discuss, but it is crucial for your overall care and quality of life to discuss issues beyond the physical ones with your HCP. Any personal problems in other domains of your life can have a powerful effect on your physical health. As seen in **Figure 1**, when an individual is sick or has a chronic illness this affects all aspects of their quality of life. If you are honest and discuss physical, psychological, social, and spiritual issues, then all decisions about your health will be made while taking into account what will positively increase your quality of life.

97. If I have ongoing health problems and I am feeling anxious or down should I tell my HCP?

You should always discuss your emotional state with your HCP.

It is normal for all individuals to have periods in their lives when they feel sad or anxious or depressed. Sometimes it is due to a specific situation (e.g., a loss of a job, or the death of a family member). But you can also experience many different psychological or emotional feelings when you have ongoing or chronic health problems (see Figure 1). This is normal. You should always discuss your emotional state with your HCP. Your HCP can help you figure out which feelings are normal reactions and help you decide which coping mechanisms to use.

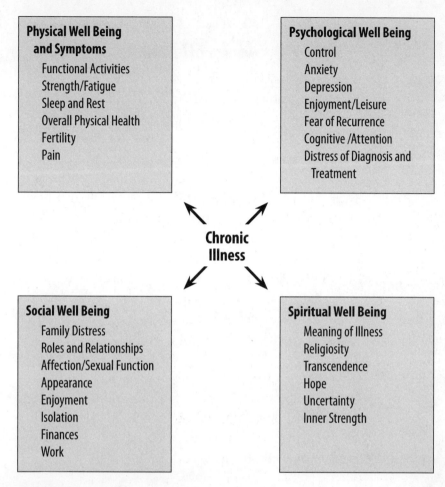

Figure 1 Quality of Life and Chronic Illness

You must be honest with your HCP and let him or her know if you have considered suicide. Your HCP can also help by making a referral to a psychologist (to talk about what you are going through) or psychiatrist (for medications to help you through this tough period) or a social worker (to help with community referrals). The **social worker** can help you locate support groups in your area or help you develop new coping mechanisms.

You must be honest with your HCP and let him or her know if you have considered suicide.

98. Should I tell my HCP if my illness is affecting my social life?

Frequently individuals with chronic illnesses start treatments recommended by their HCP and begin to feel better physically, but the illness and treatment may be seriously affecting their social lives

Frequently individuals with chronic illnesses start treatments recommended by their HCP and begin to feel better physically, but the illness and treatment may be seriously affecting their social lives (see Figure 1). In terms of family life, when one family member develops a chronic health problem it can significantly affect the roles and responsibilities of all of the family members. For example, if the mother of four children develops a chronic illness that is being treated but leaves her feeling fatigued, she may not be able to do all the chores she did before. Thus, the father and the children's roles may change, and they may have to take on new responsibilities. The mother's condition may further affect the family socially if she was working part-time and has to take a leave of absence; then this will lead to a decrease in income. Or the mother may continue to work part-time, but between working and her treatment she may be too tired to attend school activities with her children (e.g., sports games, theater, PTA). And the mother may become isolated from friends.

99. Should I tell my HCP if my illness is affecting my spiritual life?

It is vital to tell your HCP if you are experiencing spiritual distress from your illness because this can ultimately affect you physically, psychologically, and socially.

As human beings we are all spiritual. Some individuals may not be religious and that is fine. But everyone has a spirit and a soul. When an individual has a chronic illness it can affect his/her spiritual well-being and ultimately his/her quality of life (see Figure 1). Again, it is vital to tell your HCP if you are experiencing spiritual distress from your illness because this can ultimately affect you physically, psychologically, and socially. Some individuals with health problems actually experience an increase in spiritual well-being and/or increase in faith/religion. For other individuals there is distress and a feeling of hopelessness, a feeling of uncertainty about the future, and a questioning of the meaning of their life.

100. Where can I find more information?

It used to be that patients automatically took the advice of their HCP without a second thought. Today, more and more individuals are getting involved in managing their health. One way to do this is to actively research your illness and treatment options. First, determine your goals for conducting the research. For instance, you may want to find out what the standard treatment is for your illness, or who are the top HCPs or top treatment centers for your specific illness, or learn about complementary therapies.

To start gathering medical information it is best to buy a good medical dictionary. Look at several before you buy one. Some have illustrations or larger print for ease of reading. Whatever your diagnosis, *The Merck Manual of Diagnosis and Therapy* will explain it thoroughly. This is in more technical language, but you can find this book at the library or go to the Internet at *www.merck.com*. This explains causes, symptoms, tests, diagnosis, treatment, and prognosis. Additionally, Merck has recently released a lay version called the *Merck Manual of Medical Information: Home Edition*.

To start gathering medical information it is best to buy a good medical dictionary.

Many individuals find it helpful to contact support organizations or foundations. Many of these organizations are listed in the Appendix of this book. Whether you go to a local office or an Internet site, organizations can provide information, support groups, newsletters, journals, and book reviews regarding illnesses and treatments.

Despite all the technological advantages, public libraries are still very useful. There are also medical and university libraries. Libraries can provide books, journals, newspapers, and computers.

Lastly, the Internet is increasingly becoming the most up-to-date source of comprehensive information on illnesses and treatments. The Appendix provides an extensive list of resources for patients and families. Almost all of these resources have a website listed. Each of these Internet sites can be considered a credible healthcare resource. There are also Internet sites that have been created by one or two patients or groups of lay people or promotional sites. The information on these sites may not be credible or accurate.

Appendix

AboutFace USA

www.aboutfaceusa.org

AboutFace USA is a nonprofit organization dedicated to providing information, emotional support, and educational programs to individuals who have a facial disfigurement, and to their families.

AIM Doc Finder

State Medical Board Executive Directors

www.docboard.org

This is an online resource sponsored by a nonprofit organization providing access to a health professional database.

Alpha-1 Foundation

www.alphaone.org

The Alpha-1 Foundation is dedicated to providing the leadership and resources that will result in increased research, improved health, worldwide detection and a cure for Alpha-1 Antitrypsin Deficiency (Alpha-1). Alpha-1 is a genetic disorder that can cause liver and lung disease in children and adults.

Alstrom Syndrome International

www.jax.org/alstrom

The mission of Alstrom Syndrome International is to provide support and information, and to coordinate world-wide with families and professionals in order to treat and cure Alstrom Syndrome.

Alzheimer's Association, Inc.

www.alz.org

The mission of the Alzheimer's Association is to eliminate Alzheimer's disease through the advancement of research and to enhance quality care and support for individuals, their families, and care partners.

AMA Physician Select

American Medical Association
515 North State Street
Chicago, IL 60610
(800) 621-8335
www.ama-assn.org

AMA database of demographic and professional information on individual physicians in the United States.

American Academy on Communication in Healthcare

www.aachonline.org

AACH fosters the best patient care by advocating a relationship-centered approach to healthcare communication, education, and research.

American Academy of Home Care Physicians at 410-676-7966

www.aahcp.org

Since 1988, the American Academy of Home Care Physicians has served the needs of thousands of physicians and related professionals and agencies interested in improving care of patients in the home.

American Autoimmune Related Diseases Association

www.aarda.org

The American Autoimmune Related Diseases Association is dedicated to the eradication of autoimmune diseases and the alleviation of suffering and the socioeconomic impact of autoimmunity through fostering and facilitating collaboration in the areas of education, public awareness, research, and patient services in an effective, ethical, and efficient manner.

American Brain Tumor Association

www.abta.org

The American Brain Tumor Association exists to eliminate brain tumors through research and to meet the needs of brain tumor patients and their families.

American Board of Medical Specialties
1007 Church Street, Suite 404
Evanston, IL 60201
(866) ASK-ABMS
(847) 491-9091
www.abms.org

ABMS provides verification of physician qualifications and list of individual specialties. After registering on the Website, click on the "who's certified" button and search by physician name or specialty.

American Cancer Society
1599 Clifton Road, NE
Atlanta, GA 30329
(800) ACS·2345
www.cancer.org

The American Cancer Society (ACS) is a nationwide, community-based voluntary health organization. Headquartered in Atlanta, Georgia, the ACS has state divisions and more than 3,400 local offices.

American Diabetes Association
www.diabetes.org

The American Diabetes Association is the nation's leading non-profit health organization providing diabetes research, information and advocacy. The mission of the Association is to prevent and cure diabetes and to improve the lives of all people affected by diabetes.

American Heart Association
www.americanheart.org

The American Heart Association is a national voluntary health agency whose mission is to reduce disability and death from cardiovascular diseases and stroke.

American Kidney Fund

www.kidneyfund.org

The American Kidney Fund is the nation's leading voluntary health organization serving people with and at risk for kidney disease through direct financial assistance, comprehensive education, clinical research, and community service programs.

American Liver Foundation

www.liverfoundation.org

The American Liver Foundation (ALF) is a national nonprofit organization dedicated to the prevention, treatment, and cure of hepatitis and other liver diseases through research, education, and advocacy on behalf of those at risk or affected by liver disease.

American Lung Association

www.lungusa.org

The American Lung Association fights lung disease in all its forms, with special emphasis on asthma, tobacco control, and environmental health.

American Skin Association

www.americanskin.org

The American Skin Association (ASA) is a volunteer-led health organization dedicated—through research, education, and advocacy—to saving lives and alleviating human suffering caused by the full spectrum of skin disorders.

American Tinnitus Association

www.ata.org

The American Tinnitus Association (ATA) is the national champion of tinnitus awareness, prevention, and treatment.

American Urologic Association Foundation

(formerly American Foundation of Urologic Disease)

www.auafoundation.org

The mission of the American Urologic Foundation is the prevention and cure of urologic diseases through the expansion of research, education, and patient advocacy.

Arthritis Foundation

www.arthritis.org

The mission of the Arthritis Foundation is to improve lives through leadership in the prevention, control, and cure of arthritis and related diseases.

Asthma and Allergy Foundation of American

www.aafa.org

The Asthma and Allergy Foundation of America (AAFA) is the premier patient organization dedicated to improving the quality of life for people with asthma and allergies and other caregivers, through education, advocacy, and research.

BCCNS Life Support Network

www.bccns.org

The BCCNS Life Support Network supports people and families affected by Basal Cell Carcinoma Syndrome through education, referrals, support, and research.

Best Hospitals Finder (*U.S. News and World Report*)

health.usnews.com/sections/health/best-hospitals

The U.S. News hospital rankings are designed to assist patients in their search for the highest level of medical care. Database is searchable by specialty.

Brain Injury Association of America

www.biausa.org

The Brain Injury Association of America's mission is to create a better future through brain injury prevention, research, education, and advocacy.

Celiac Sprue Association/USA

www.csaceliacs.org

As a member-based, nonprofit organization, Celiac Sprue Association (CSA) is dedicated to helping individuals with celiac disease and dermatitis herpetiformis and their families worldwide through education, information, and research.

Center for Medicare and Medicaid Services

7500 Security Blvd.
Baltimore, MD 21244-1850
(800) 633-4227
(866) 226-1819 (TTY)
www.cms.hhs.gov

The CMS provides extensive information and referral information on Medicaid and Medicare, including individual states' plans and how to apply.

Center for Nutrition Policy and Promotion (CNPP)

3101 Park Center Drive, Room 1034
Alexandria. VA 22302-1594
(703) 305-7600
www.usda.gov/cnpp

Provides information on general nutrition-related topics

CenterWatch
Thomson CenterWatch
22 Thomson Place, 47F1
Boston, MA 02210-1212
Phone: (617) 856-5900
Fax: (617) 856-5901
www.centerwatch.com
Provides a listing of clinical trials

Children and Adults with Attention Deficit/Hyperactivity Disorder (CHADD)
www.chadd.org
CHADD works to improve the lives of people affected by AD/HD through collaborative leadership, advocacy, research, education, and support.

Chromosome Deletion Outreach, Inc.
www.chromodisorder.org
Chromosome Deletion Outreach's mission is to provide support to parents of children born with rare chromosome disorders, gather and disseminate information, and promote research and a positive community understanding of these disorders.

Central Nervous System Vasculitis Foundation (CSNV)
www.cnsvfinc.org
CNSV-network is a patient-centered, non-commercial, volunteer-run website and Internet-based support service for people with Central Nervous System Vasculitis, their families, and the health-care community.

Cutaneous Lymphoma Foundation
www.clfoundation.org
The Cutaneous Lymphoma Foundation is an independent, non-profit patient advocacy organization dedicated to supporting people with cutaneous lymphomas by promoting awareness and education, advancing patient care, and facilitating research.

Department of Veterans Affairs

Veterans Health Association
810 Vermont Avenue, NW
Washington, DC 20420
(800) 827-1000 (local Virginia office)
(202) 273-5400 (Washington, DC office)
www.va.gov

This site provides extensive information for veterans. It is a one-stop site for all concerns regarding veterans' benefits and services. Eligibility forms can be either downloaded or completed online.

Easter Seals

www.easterseals.com

Easter Seals has been helping individuals with disabilities and special needs, and their families, live better lives for more than 80 years.

Epilepsy Foundation

www.epilepsyfoundation.org

The Epilepsy Foundation will ensure that people with seizures are able to participate in all life experiences; and will prevent, control, and cure epilepsy through research, education, advocacy, and services.

Families of Spinal Muscular Dystrophy

www.fsma.org

Families of Spinal Muscular Atrophy is the largest international organization dedicated solely to eradicating spinal muscular atrophy (SMA) by promoting and supporting research; helping families cope with SMA through informational programs and support; and educating the public and professional community about SMA.

Health Resources and Services Administration (HRSA)
Hill-Burton program
U.S. Department of Health and Human Services Administration
Parklawn Building
5600 Fishers Lane
Rockville, MD 20857
(800) 638-0742
(301) 443-5656
(800) 492-0359 (from the Maryland area)
www.hrsa.gov

Site provides information on many government initiatives and programs related to providing health care to low income and disadvantaged populations.

Huntington's Disease Society of America
www.hdsa.org

The Huntington's Disease Society of America (HDSA) is dedicated to finding a cure for Huntington's Disease (HD) while providing support and services for those living with HD and their families.

International Mosaic Down Syndrome Association
www.imdsa.com

International Mosaic Down Syndrome Association is designed to provide emotional support, information and research to those touched by Mosaic Down Syndrome.

International Pemphigus Foundation
www.pemphigus.org

The International Pemphigus Foundation is dedicated to providing information and support to the community of people living with the rare autoimmune skin disease pemphigus and phemphigoid, including the family members, friends, and medical professionals who care for them.

International Rett Syndrome Association

www.rettsyndrome.org

The mission of the International Rett Syndrome Association (IRSA) is to support and stimulate biomedical research that will determine the cause and find treatments and cures for Rett Syndrome, to increase public awareness of Rett syndrome, and to provide informational and emotional support to families of children with Rett Syndrome.

Interstitial Cystitis Association

www.ichelp.com

Founded in 1984, the Interstitial Cystitis Foundation (ICA) is a not-for-profit health organization dedicated to providing patient and physician educational information and programs, patient support, public awareness and, most importantly, research funding.

Kidney Cancer Association

www.curekidneycancer.org

The Kidney Cancer Association is a membership organization made up of patients, family members, physicians, researchers, and other health professionals.

Lance Armstrong Foundation

www.laf.org

The Lance Armstrong Foundation (LAF) believes that in the battle with cancer, knowledge is power and attitude is everything. Founded in 1997 by cancer survivor and cycling champion Lance Armstrong, the LAF provides the practical information and tools people living with cancer need to live strong.

Language Line Services
1 Lower Ragsdale Drive
Building 2
Monterey, CA 93490
(877) 886-3885
www.languageline.com

The "Personal Interpreter" is a pay-as-you-go service that allows you to access interpreters in more than 140 languages from any phone 24/7, 365 days a year. There is a fee to use these services if your hospital does not have a contract with the company; you can use a credit card to pay. The website also provides a description of the services provided including document translation.

Law Help
www.lawhelp.org

An online legal and lawyer referral service for people with low or moderate income.

The web site is run by a nonprofit organization based in New York City, but has information through partner organizations in many other states.

Lupus Foundation of America, Inc.
www.lupus.org

With more than 200 chapters, branches and support groups in 30 states, the Lupus Foundation of America (LFA) is the nation's leading nonprofit voluntary health organization dedicated to finding the causes and cure of lupus. Their mission is to improve the diagnosis and treatment of lupus, support individuals and families affected by the disease, increase awareness of lupus among health professionals and the public, and find the causes and cure.

Meals on Wheels
1414 Prince Street, Suite 302
Alexandria, VA 22314
(703) 548-5588
www.mowaa.org

This organization provides home-delivered meals to those in need, such as people who have trouble grocery shopping or cooking their own food. The web site allows you to search for local programs.

The Merck Manual of Diagnosis and Therapy explains causes, symptoms, tests, diagnosis, treatment and prognosis of almost any illness. This book is in more technical language, but you can find this book at the library or go to the Internet at *www.merck.com*. Additionally, Merck has recently released a lay version called the *Merck Manual of Medical Information: Home Edition.*

My Personal Health Record
www.myPHR.com

A guide to understanding and managing your personal health information, this web site is provided as a free public service by the American Health Information Management Association (AHIMA). The AHIMA is a national nonprofit professional association dedicated to the effective management of personal health information needed to deliver quality health care to the public.

Myasthenia Gravis Foundation of America, Inc.
www.myasthenia.org

The Mission of the Foundation is to facilitate the timely diagnosis and optimal care of individuals affected by myasthenia gravis and closely related disorders and to improve their lives through programs of patient services, public information, medical research, professional education, advocacy, and patient care.

National Alopecia Areata Foundation

www.naaf.org

The mission of the National Alopecia Areata Foundation (NAAF) is to support research to find a cure or acceptable treatment for alopecia areata, to support those with the disease and to education the public about alopecia areata.

National Aphasia Association

www.aphasia.org

The National Aphasia Association (NAA) is a nonprofit organization that promotes public education, research, rehabilitation, and support services to assist people with aphasia and their families.

National Cancer Institute (Clinical Trials)

1-800-4-CANCER

www.cancer.gov/clinicaltrials

Provides information specifically related to clinical trials for cancer

National Center for Complementary and Alternative Medicine

NCCAM Clearinghouse
Post Office Box7923
Gaithersburg, MD 20898
(888) 644-6226
www.ncam.nih.gov

This site provides information regarding disease-specific alternatives and complementary therapies. The site covers the basics on using these therapies, where to find doctors, research, and clinical trials all related to complementary and alternative medicine. Some information is available in Spanish.

The National Council on the Aging

300 D Street, SW, Suite 801
Washington, DC 20024
(202) 479-1200
(202) 479-6674 (TDD)
www.ncoa.org

This is a nonprofit organization focusing on informing the older consumer regarding all types of medical issues. The site provides a list of resources and publications that are specifically designed to help older individuals cope with various health issues and offers a Benefits Checkup tool that screens seniors' eligibility for benefits programs.

National Down Syndrome Society

www.ndss.org

The mission of the National Down Syndrome Society is to benefit people with Down Syndrome and their families through national leadership in education, research, and advocacy.

National Eczema Association

www.nationaleczema.org

The National Eczema Association for Science and Education (NEASE) works to improve the health and the quality of life of all persons living with atopic dermatitis/eczema, providing emotional support, information, and resources to those who have the disease, as well as their loved ones, while raising public awareness of the disease.

National Family Caregivers Association (NFCA)

10400 Connecticut Avenue, Suite 500
Kensington, MD 20895-3944
(800) 896-3650
www.nfcacares.org

Espousing a philosophy of self-advocacy and self-care, the NFCA provides a variety of educational materials (available through their website) to support family caregivers.

National Hemophilia Foundation

www.hemophilia.org

The mission of the National Hemophilia Foundation is education, research and advocacy on behalf of people with bleeding disorders.

National Hospice and Palliative Care Organization (NHPCO)

1700 Diagonal Road, Suite 625
Alexandria, VA 22314
(800) 658-8898
www.nhpco.org

Provides information on hospice services nationally, including information on communication about hospice, insurance coverage, and locating hospice services. The organization provides explanations of palliative care, Medicare benefits, and other frequently asked questions. Information is also available in Spanish.

National Kidney Foundation

www.kidney.org

The National Kidney Foundation, Inc., a major voluntary health organization, seeks to prevent kidney and urinary tract diseases, improve the health and well-being of individuals and families affected by these diseases, and increase the availability of all organs for transplantation.

National Marfan Foundation

www.marfan.org

The National Marfan Foundation is dedicated to saving lives, and improving the quality of life for individuals and families affected by the Marfan Syndrome and related disorders.

National Marrow Donor Program

www.marrow.org

The National Marrow Donor Program (NMDP) helps people who need a life-saving marrow or blood cell transplant. They connect patients, doctors, donors and researchers to resources they need to help more people live longer, healthier lives.

National Mental Health Association

www.nmha.org

The National Mental Health Association is dedicated to promoting mental health, preventing mental disorders and achieving victory over mental illness through advocacy, education, research, and service.

National Multiple Sclerosis Society

www.nmss.org

The mission of the National Multiple Sclerosis Society is to end the devastating effects of multiple sclerosis.

National Osteoporosis Foundation

www.nof.org

The National Osteoporosis Foundation's mission is to prevent osteoporosis, to promote lifelong bone health, to help improve the lives of those affected by osteoporosis and related fractures, and to find a cure.

National Ovarian Cancer Coalition

www.ovarian.org

The mission of the National Ovarian Cancer Coalition is to raise awareness and promote education about ovarian cancer. The Coalition is committed to improving the survival rate and quality of life for women with ovarian cancer.

National Pediculosis Association, Inc.

www.headlice.org

The National Pediculosis Association®, Inc. (NPA) is the only nonprofit health and education agency dedicated to protecting children from the misuse and abuse of potentially harmful live and scabies pesticidal treatments. As part of its mission, the NPA works to encourage our nation's health and child care professionals to adopt standardized head lice management programs in an effort to keep the children in school lice and nit free.

National Psoriasis Foundation

www.psoriasis.org

The mission of the National Psoriasis Foundation is to improve the quality of life of people who have psoriasis and psoriatic arthritis. Through education and advocacy, they promote awareness and understanding, ensure access to treatment, and support research that will lead to effective management and, ultimately, a cure.

National Sleep Foundation

www.sleepfoundation.org

The National Sleep Foundation (NSF) is an independent nonprofit organization dedicated to improving public health and safety by achieving understanding of sleep and sleep disorders, and by supporting education, sleep-related research, and advocacy.

National Tay-Sachs and Allied Diseases Association

www.ntsad.org

The National Tay-Sachs and Allied Diseases Association (NTSAD) is dedicated to the treatment and prevention of Tay-Sachs, Canavan, and related genetic diseases, and to providing information and support services to individuals and families affected by these diseases, as well as to the public at large.

Needy Meds, Inc.

Post Office Box 63716
Philadelphia, PA 19147
(215) 625-9609
www.needymeds.com

Offers information about programs sponsored by pharmaceutical manufacturers to help people who cannot afford to purchase necessary drugs.

New LifeStyles Online
4144 N. Central Expressway, Suite 1000
Dallas, TX 75204
(800) 869-9549
www.newlifestyles.com

Provides information on independent retirement communities, assisted living, nursing homes, Alzheimer's care, and home or hospice care. You can order a free guide or search online.

Pancreatic Cancer Action Network
www.pancan.org

The pancreatic Cancer Action Network, Inc. (PanCAN), established in 1999, is the first national patient advocacy organization for the pancreatic cancer community. PanCAN works to focus national attention on the need to find a cure for pancreatic cancer.

Parent Project Muscular Dystrophy
www.parentprojectmd.org

Parent Project Muscular Dystrophy's mission is to improve the treatment, quality of life, and long-term outlook for all individuals affected by Duchenne and Becker Muscular Dystrophy.

Polycystic Ovarian Syndrome Association
www.pcosupport.org

The Polycystic Ovarian Syndrome Association exists to provide comprehensive information, support, and advocacy for women and girls with the condition known as polycystic ovary syndrome.

Prevent Blindness America
www.preventblindness.org

Founded in 1908, Prevent Blindness America is the nation's leading volunteer eye health and safety organization dedicated to fighting blindness and saving sight.

Social Security Administration (SSA)
Office of Public Inquiries
Windsor Park Building
6401 Security Blvd
Baltimore, MD 21235
(800) 772-1213
(800) 325-0778 (TTY)
www.ssa.gov

This Federal program provides extensive information on Social Security Benefits including Social Security Disability (SSD), Medicare, Supplementary Security Income (SSI), contact information to state Medicaid offices, and much more. You may be able to apply online to these programs, and even check your claim status. Information is available in many languages; call or check the website for a complete list.

U.S. Department of Health and Human Services
200 Independence Avenue
Washington, DC 20201
(877) 696-6775
www.hhs.gov

The mission of this government organization is to "protect health and give a special helping hand to those who need assistance." HHS provides information on many topics including Medicare, Medicaid, childcare and health initiatives, referrals to information on cancer, and much more. HHS publishes the "Guide to Health Insurance for People with Medicare."

U. S. Department of Labor
Frances Perkins Building
200 Constitution Avenue, NW
Washington, DC 20210
(866) 4-USA-DOL
www.dol.gov/esa/whd/fmla

The U.S. Department of Labor has created an online program to help people understand their eligibility for and rights regarding the Family Medical Act. Additional information regarding employee rights, including health plans and benefits, is available in the e-laws section of the website.

Glossary

A

Advanced directives: Legal documents in which you indicate who you want to make medical decisions for you and/or what type of medical treatments you want to receive if you become unable to make decisions or speak for yourself.

B

Billing Clerk: An individual who is responsible for compiling and maintaining records of the charges for services rendered at the healthcare facility. Once they calculate the total amount due from a patient, they must prepare invoices to be sent out and ensure prompt payment.

C

Cardiologist: Physician who specializes in heart problems.

Clinical trials: Research studies conducted to test the effectiveness of new treatments on human beings.

Colonoscopy: Examination of the large intestine with a fiberoptic instrument. It allows the physician to look for inflammatory problems, polyps or tumors. This technique allows for specimens to be taken. A baseline colonoscopy is recommended for everyone at age 50 to help screen for colorectal cancer.

Colorectal surgeon: Performs surgery on the intestinal tract, colon, rectum, and organs affected by the intestine.

Complementary medicine or **therapies:** Healing treatment(s) used together with mainstream, hospital-based medical practice.

Complete blood count (CBC): A blood test to measure the number of white blood cells, red blood cells, and platelets.

Computed tomography (CT) Scan: A special X-ray study that takes pictures of the inside of your body. A narrow X-ray beam moves around a section of your body. The images produced are patterned much like a slice of bread. These pictures are made to focus on the body part(s) your doctor needs to see (e.g., abdomen).

Consultants (or specialists): Healthcare providers other than your primary HCP who are asked to give an opinion about your condition.

D

Doctor of Osteopathy (DO): Has a Doctors degree in Osteopathy, which is a system of medicine based on the theory that disturbances in the musculoskeletal system affect other bodily parts, causing many disorders that can be corrected by various manipulative techniques in conjunction with conventional medical, surgical, pharmacological, and other therapeutic procedures.

Do not resuscitate (DNR) orders: Indication in a patients medical chart based on the expressed wishes of the patient or their healthcare proxy that no extraordinary life-extending measures are to be taken if they stop breathing or their heart stops beating.

E

Elder abuse includes the following types: **Physical abuse** is the infliction of bodily injury and may be manifested by lacerations, fractures, soft tissue trauma, burns or bruises. **Sexual abuse** is any form of intimate sexual activity without consent. **Emotional or psychological abuse** is the infliction of mental anguish, such as intimidation by yelling, insulting, threatening, or silence. **Financial exploitation** is the misuse of another persons funds or assets without his or her explicit knowledge or consent. **Caregiver neglect** is the malicious neglect by a caregiver of an older persons needs, whether for retaliation, disinterest, or financial incentives.

F

Family Practitioner: A physician who specializes in caring for all the family members (e.g., babies to adults).

G

General surgeon: A physician who performs operations of many different types. But, there are also subspecialists in surgery.

Geriatrician: A physician who specializes in the medical care of older people (e.g., >60 or 65 years old).

Geriatrics: The department of medicine or dentistry that treats health problems peculiar to advanced age and the aging, including the clinical problems of senescence and senility.

Gerontology: The scientific study of old age.

Gynecologist: A physician who specializes in womens health.

H

Healthcare proxy: A person designated to make healthcare decisions for you if you are not able to do so; also called a healthcare surrogate, a medical proxy, or a medical power of attorney.

Hematocrit: The proportion of blood which is red blood cells; expressed as a percentage; used as a measure of the amount of red blood cells.

Hemoglobin: Substance in red blood cells that binds to oxygen and carries it to tissues of the body; used as a measure of the amount of red blood cells.

Herbal therapies: Individual herbs or mixtures of herbs that are used for therapeutic value.

Home care: Medical, nursing, social, or rehabilitative services provided in the patients home.

Hospice: A philosophy of care that helps you live the rest of your life with quality and dignity and to be symptom-free when your life expectancy is 6 months or less.

I

Informed consent: Means that you understand and give permission for a treatment, procedure or medication, even though there may be benefits and complications.

Internist: A physician who specializes in the diagnosis and medical treatment of adults.

L

Licensed Practical Nurse (LPN): A nurse who has a two-year degree in nursing and is limited in the care they can provide under the direction of an RN, NP, PA or MD.

Living Will: Document in which you can state specific instructions regarding your health care, including measures that would prolong your life; it

may also outline which medical interventions you want to have withheld for a variety of circumstances.

M

Magnetic Resonance Imaging (MRI) Scan: Test which uses magnetic and low energy radio waves to produce a series of pictures. It does not use any type of X-ray beam. It is important to tell your HCP of any surgeries or accidents that may have left metal clips or objects in your body.

Mammography: Use of an X-ray image of the breasts on photographic film to detect cancers that may not be discovered by breast self-exam or the clinical exam of a HCP. Generally, women should have a baseline mammogram at age 40. If there is a family history of breast cancer, then you may need a mammogram at an earlier age.

Medicaid: A medical benefits program administered by states and subsidized by the federal government. Under this plan, various medical expenses will be paid to those who qualify. It is technically referred to as Title XIX Benefits.

Medicare: A federal health insurance program.

Medigap: A form of private supplementary insurance.

Minerals: Nutrients needed by the body in small amounts to help it function properly and stay strong.

Iron, calcium, potassium, and sodium are minerals.

N

Neurologist: A physician who takes care of people who have problems or diseases of the nervous system.

Neurosurgeon: A physician who specializes in surgery of the brain, brain stem, skull, spine, spinal cord, and nerves.

Nurse Practitioner (NP): A registered nurse (RN) with a masters degree who has completed additional courses and specialized training. Nurse practitioners can work with or without the supervision of a physician. They take on additional duties in diagnosis and treatment of patients, and in most states they write all types of prescriptions.

O

Oncologist: A physician who specializes in treating cancer; **surgical oncologists** specialize in cancer surgery; **medical oncologists** specialize in treatment with chemotherapy, hormonal therapy, and biologic therapy; **radiation oncologists** specialize in treating with radiation.

P

Pediatric surgeon: A physician who operates on children, from newborns to teenagers.

Pediatrician: A physician who specializes in the care of babies and children up to about age 16–18 years old.

Physician (MD): A licensed medical practitioner, a person who practices medicine, a person licensed by the jurisdiction in which he/she is resident as a medical doctor to practice the healing arts.

Physician Assistant (PA): A trained, licensed individual who can diagnose, treat, and write prescriptions under the direction of a supervising physician.

Platelets: Blood cells that help prevent bleeding by causing clots to form when a blood vessel is cut; also called thrombocytes.

Q

Quality of Life: Generally thought to be comprised of four domains including physical well-being, psychological well-being, social well-being, and spiritual well-being.

R

Receptionist: An individual who answers the telephone, receives patients, checks insurance, and checks appointments in a doctor's office. This is an office/administrative support position and is usually performed in a front office.

Red blood cells: Cells in the blood that contain hemoglobin which carries oxygen from the lungs to all the tissues in the body, also called erythrocytes.

Registered Nurse (RN): A nurse who has graduated from a formal program of nursing education (diploma school, associate degree or baccalaureate program) and is registered and licensed by the appropriate state authority.

S

Secretary: An individual who works in an office/administrative support position. The title refers to a person who performs routine, administrative tasks for the doctor, NP, and/or PA. These office employees perform duties such as typing, computer processing, and transcription of dictation.

Social workers: Professionals who are trained, certified, and licensed to talk with people and their families about emotional or physical needs, and to find them support services.

U

Ultrasound: A test that uses sound waves to produce images of organs inside your body. No X-rays or radiation are used in this test.

Urologist: A doctor who specializes in problems or diseases of the urinary tract.

V

Vascular surgeon: A physician who performs surgery on disorders of the blood vessels.

Vitamins: Organic substances required to regulate the proper functioning of cells. Vitamins are either fat-soluble (vitamin E, vitamin A, vitamin D, and vitamin K) or they are water-soluble (vitamin C and the B vitamins). Vitamins are essential to life. Research now confirms the benefits of vitamins (specifically vitamin C and vitamin E) for the proper functioning and protection of the external body. Vitamin C, vitamin E, and vitamin B are formulated in EC Mode Hair and Scalp Care Systems. Vitamin C and vitamin E are formulated in EC Mode Skin Care Systems.

White blood cells: Cells in the blood that fight off infection and other types of disease; also called leukocytes. There are many different types of white blood cells that include neutrophils and lymphocytes.

Index

Italicized page locators indicate a figure; tables are noted with a *t*.